## Advance Praise for Holly Bellebuono:

"A cornucopia of herbal insights blended with the practical skills to bring nature's healing gifts into family life."—David Hoffmann, BSc, FNIMH, medical herbalist

# an Herbalist's
# GUIDE to FORMULARY

## About the Author

An American medical herbalist of twenty-three years, Holly Bellebuono is renowned for her work documenting women healers and teaching herbal formulary and pharmacology. Holly's seven-year project of interviews and research culminated in the documentary book *Women Healers of the World: The Traditions, History & Geography of Herbal Medicine* and was awarded Book of the Year by the International Herb Association and the Gold Award for Women's Books by Nautilus Book Awards. Holly directs the Bellebuono School of Herbal Medicine on Martha's Vineyard, training and certifying community herbalists in herbal medicine, and she is the founder of Vineyard Herbs Teas & Apothecary. Her work has been featured in *Parabola, SageWoman, Juno* (Britain), *Taproot, The New York Times*, and more, and her four other books include *The Essential Herbal for Natural Health, The Authentic Herbal Healer, Goal Setting for Open-Minded Business Owners*, and *The Healing Kitchen*. As a two-time Small Business Owner of the Year Award recipient, Holly leads empowerment seminars for entrepreneurs, and she facilitates seminars, retreats, and lectures for women's and business conferences and universities about herbal medicine, symbolism, and the philosophy of healing. Holly lives on Martha's Vineyard with her family; you can learn more about her work or enroll in her school at www.HollyBellebuono.com.

# HOLLY BELLEBUONO

# an Herbalist's
# GUIDE to FORMULARY

## The Art & Science of Creating
## Effective Herbal Remedies

Llewellyn Publications
Woodbury, Minnesota

FIRST EDITION
Seventh Printing, 2024

Book design by Bob Gaul
Cover design by Kevin R. Brown
Editing by Aaron Lawrence

Llewellyn Publications is a registered trademark of Llewellyn Worldwide Ltd.

**Library of Congress Cataloging-in-Publication Data**
The Library of Congress has already cataloged an earlier printing under LCCN: 2017035201

Llewellyn Worldwide Ltd. does not participate in, endorse, or have any authority or responsibility concerning private business transactions between our authors and the public.

All mail addressed to the author is forwarded, but the publisher cannot, unless specifically instructed by the author, give out an address or phone number.

Any Internet references contained in this work are current at publication time, but the publisher cannot guarantee that a specific location will continue to be maintained. Please refer to the publisher's website for links to authors' websites and other sources.

Llewellyn Publications
A Division of Llewellyn Worldwide Ltd.
2143 Wooddale Drive
Woodbury, MN 55125-2989
www.llewellyn.com

Printed in the United States of America

# Other Books by the Author

*The Healing Kitchen: Cooking with Nourishing Herbs for Health, Wellness and Vitality.* Roost Books/Shambhala Publishers, 2016.

*Women Healers of the World: The Traditions, History & Geography of Herbal Medicine.* SkyHorse Publishers, 2014.

*The Essential Herbal for Natural Health: How to Transform Easy-to-Find Herbs into Healing Remedies for the Whole Family.* Roost Books/Shambhala Publishers, 2012.

*The Authentic Herbal Healer: The Complete Guide to Herbal Formulary & Plant-Inspired Medicine for Every Body System.* Balboa, 2012.

*A Goal-Setting Guide for Open-Minded Business Owners.* A brainstorming workbook, 2015.

*How to Use Herbs for Natural Health.* Audio CD series, 2011.

# Dedication

This book is gratefully dedicated to all the women and men I've studied with, learned from, and who have shared this wonderful tradition with me.

# Acknowledgments

Many thanks to my wonderful agent, Jody Kahn, for her tireless and encouraging support; it is much appreciated! And thanks to my dad, Bill Horton, for his enthusiastic enjoyment of chemistry, biology, and inspiring his kids.

# Health Disclaimer

The information included here is for educational purposes only; it reflects the author's experience and is not intended as a substitute for professional medical care. If you are sick or injured, please seek the advice of a trusted health care professional.

# Contents

# Introduction:
# Wholeness and the Ultimate Question–
# What Is Healing?

In my twenty-three years as an herbalist dispensing medicines and supporting clients, I've been called a healer, though for decades I considered myself more of a facilitator. When customers used my apothecary products and reported back that the first-aid ointment healed their terrible burn, or the sedative tincture gave them their first solid sleep through the night, they claimed I healed them, and I quickly pointed out that it wasn't me, it was the plants. For a long time I was loath to accept any credit for the good works of my products, but over the years I've explored the interconnections between myself, the plants, my products, and the people who come to me sick, injured, or concerned, and I've questioned: when they get better, what, exactly, was my role in their recovery?

Is healing a process or an outcome? Is it scientific or personal? Who has the ability and the authority to heal—and who doesn't? In other words, what does it mean to be a healer? This is one of the deepest and most important questions we can ask ourselves as healing arts professionals, and it's a difficult and even controversial one to answer. It has become vogue to say that we can create our own health, or even that we can influence or change our reality through positive thinking. I think this is both true and untrue. I believe our thoughts have a direct impact on our lives, and they can even structure the energy that makes up our existence with direct cause-and-effect. But I've worked with enough positive people who have faced illness despite their positive mindset. People who eat well, live happily, and promote a positive ideology can still get sick and die. This begs a lot of questions: What causes illness? What causes health? And who, ultimately, is the healer?

For far too long, sick people have relied on the medical establishment to provide healing. It has been assumed that the educated physician heals with every prescription written. But do doctors heal? Does healing come from an educated mind and a prescription pad?

What about other healing arts practitioners? Do those of us who work with plants, teach nutrition, or lead yoga classes heal? True, we facilitate the healing process and guide a sick person toward wellness, but do we heal? Do our herbs and remedies heal? If so, is it the chemical nature of the plant that brings about change in the body, or is it the inherent spiritual energy of a plant that heals? Perhaps it is the connection with Mother Nature or with a divine origin that shifts a person's health. Does healing come from prayer? Does God make a sick person better? Generations of families have relied on their religious tenets to cure the sick, regarding faith as both the curative agent and the pillar upon which to lean when healing failed. Many of the indigenous women healers I've interviewed for my documentary have attributed healing to the Divine and are adamant that we as the healers are the conduit to mysterious and powerful forces beyond our understanding.

There are as many possibilities for the origin of health as there are remedies: W as it the herbs or the hugs or the chicken soup?

We may never know the answers to these questions. But it is our responsibility, as healing arts practitioners, to consider all options and to approach our clients with the open-minded respect they deserve. Personally, I think a combination of all these forces and energies leads to changes that can bring about healing, but your own experience must come into play when you are helping a person get better. Your own attitudes, confidence (or lack thereof), and beliefs will influence the person with whom you are working, regardless of whether you prescribe an antibiotic or a homemade tincture. Evaluate yourself to determine if you are open-minded and fair, and especially if you are a good listener and not a lecturer to your patients. And, importantly, be willing to work with others in a wide range of disciplines to make sure that the person has access to as many healing techniques and providers as he or she feels necessary. Healing is, by its nature, a collaborative process, and part of our job is to facilitate the connections that will best serve the person in need.

We still face enormous mysteries in life, death, and illness; for this reason I want to address one important concept that is seldom discussed in the herbal medicine world: What happens when healing methods fail?

## Failure and Success, and Priorities for Care

Unfortunately, many people assume their goal should be perfect health. This is noble and ideal, of course—why work toward anything less? But basing self-worth (or even the worth of an entire healing tradition) on the success or failure of, say, curing cancer is not in line with the philosophies of a healing arts practitioner. No one is perfect, and to strive toward a perfect human body will only result in disappointment. It is a hard lesson: the bitter realization that we can control some things but not everything. That some people will recover and others won't. A feeling of failure can even make a person sicker than before.

Part of the problem is that many healing arts professionals believe it must mean your gift or skill as a healer is inadequate. But illness is a vastly misunderstood phenomenon, and to pin the integrity of a healing method or tradition on the basis of complete success is misguided and harmful, and it leads to the exclusion of valid healing methods (including both herbal and allopathic). I think certain priorities for healing are important for healing arts practitioners; we must ask, what is the top priority for a healer? Is it to heal? In fact, I think not.

Instead, I propose Priorities for Care, a simple list of important philosophies for the healing arts practitioner to consider that promote wholeness and connection first where the effort to solve the problem is secondary:

## Priority #1: Initiate a Relationship of Respect

Too often people express disappointment with their caregivers because they were seen quickly, spoken to hastily, and left to put their clothes back on with more questions than answers. This is a disrespectful way to treat a person seeking treatment. Respect should be the central tenet of a healing philosophy and the number one priority for any herbalist, physician, or other healer—even before "fixing the problem." Learn the person's name and go further to discover their past and their interests, diet, and goals, and open up a two-sided dialogue in which the person feels comfortable sharing private information and expressing feelings, questions, disagreements, and possible solutions.

## Priority #2: Help the Person Connect with Others

Illness can make people feel isolated and alone. By helping them connect with others, the healing arts practitioner is helping them build the bridges and networks that will sustain them through both illness and health, and this gives them a valuable resource. There are so many others who need to be in this person's network—not just you! Directly help the person contact and connect with family members, doctors, priests and rabbis, friends, counselors, therapists, other herbalists, and even help them connect with plants. Building this framework for the person who comes to you for help can be even more needed in the long run than providing a list of recommended remedies.

### Priority #3: Work to Address the Problem

Only now, after actively respecting the person and helping to establish other connections in his or her life, should the herbalist address the problem at hand. Unless you're an emergency room doctor, this step should be third on the list. And notice I don't say "fix the problem," because healing is as much in the pursuit as in the outcome. Healing arts practitioners understand the multilayered approach to healing, the levels upon which we build trust, ask questions, pursue a line of inquiry, assess a need, recommend tiers of herbs, and adjust according to need as time goes by. "Fixing" the problem is a linear thought process, but we know problems and solutions are circuitous, that life and illness and death are cyclical, and that emotions and mental health are every bit a part of the person's physical illness and must be included in the whole protocol. Working to address the problem removes this linear framework and creates an opportunity for growth and change.

Working from this priority list fits nicely into herbalism's holistic nature, and it even gives us a good basis for formulating our medicines. Knowing these priorities, we can approach formulary from the most effective and holistic perspective. Formulary is a way of structuring your thoughts to put certain herbs together, to understand their actions, and to create a healing practice that will affirm the person's needs and support the healing process. Formulary involves pharmacology, anatomy, and chemistry, as well as intuition and a connection to the person in need. It is a very creative and fulfilling endeavor; there are many ways to do it and many traditions to pull from, and our exploration of formulary will provide a strong foundation upon which the healing arts practitioner can build health.

# A Note About This Book

For the healing arts practitioner of any modality—chiropractic, acupuncture, yoga, homeopathy, nursing—herbs are an intriguing medicine. Many complementary and alternative healers as well as allopathic practitioners include, or want to include, herbs in their work, and they want to learn more about how herbs work and how to blend them into their practice. This guidebook will help the practitioner or professional navigate the complexity and depth of herbal heritage and understand how to use herbal medicine for the health of their clients and patients. As a reference, it is a straightforward list with up-to-date information about herbal chemistry and pharmacology seasoned with my personal and professional experience harvesting, processing, formulating, selling, and using herbs as medicine in a community setting.

This book features the tenets of our herbal heritage and the specifics of how to apply plant medicines in a healing capacity gleaned from my years directing an herbal retail and wholesale apothecary and a school of herbal medicine where I train and certify students in community herbalism. More and more, I meet colleagues who specialize in hands-on body healing, or I talk with physicians who are intrigued by the results they see in their patients who use herbs, and they want to learn more. This book is for you—to share what I've learned from other herbalists and healers and from my own decades as an herbalist, and especially to offer a structure in which to study the vast number of herbs in a concise and easily organized way. Many of my students have been relieved to learn how to think about formulas using the 4-tier formula I present here because it gives them a practical platform for organizing all those useful herbs. When working with a client or patient, this sensible structure helps narrow down potential remedies to those few that will be of most benefit.

Also consider that within the scope of herbal medicine is our responsibility to focus on both herbs and herbal knowledge that are garnered in a positive manner. For instance, we have the option and responsibility to purchase herbs that are organically grown or free of genetically modified organisms (GMOs)—which is not only good for the environment, but it is especially useful since many of the tier 1 tonic herbs described here will be used long-term and are meant to nourish the body; thus, acquiring pesticide-free and genetically intact herbs is vitally important. We also have the responsibility to make our voices heard about the animal testing that is, unfortunately and surprisingly, at the foundation of herbal medicine trials. Much of the scientific research being conducted about these botanicals is at the expense of animals, and while I include the results from their studies in this book, I personally and professionally do not condone such research and hope that our herbal traditions can be scientifically and clinically validated without such needless animal experimentation.

## What to Expect

While herbalism can lend itself to encyclopedic lists of herbs and their actions, it's also rich in heritage and the stories of people. This book reflects the more scientific aspects of herbal study while my book *Women Healers of the World* celebrates the more human aspect of falling in love with herbal medicine—especially through the stories of the extraordinary women throughout history who have influenced plant healing. But these are not mutually exclusive, thus, the discussion on wholeness, health, the many expectations we face as healing arts practitioners, failure or success, and thoughts about the origin of health itself are intriguing and important questions for any healer to explore.

With that discussion as our background, we will explore a brief history of healing traditions and then dive right into what I call a 4-tier formula structure. It's an easy and commonsense way to integrate a wide range of herbal actions while keeping the formula relatively small and simple—and it's what makes this book different from other herbal medicine books that may feature the history, cultivation, or use of herbs. By learning to organize herbs into effective remedies using this special formulary technique, the healing arts practitioner can call on this structure for any patient or client and with any illness or need for prevention. Be sure to refer to the five glossaries at the back of this book for detailed information about herbal chemistry, tonics, threatened and at-risk medicinal plants, and more.

Formulary is one of the most interesting and enjoyable parts of herbal medicine; up there with spending time in a sunny garden or hearing from a client that they feel better, using creative formulary is a rewarding and effective skill for the healing arts practitioner.

# PART ONE

# Formulary: Crafting Formulas in Herbal Medicine

Next to connecting with plants, formulary is at the heart of herbal education and is a key process in herbal medicine. The business of entrepreneurial herbalism, the clinical applications, even the heritage can come later, but knowing the plants intimately and learning how to combine and use them is essential. The history of formulary traditions is fascinating, and learning about the varied healing philosophies from around the world gives us an appreciation for the rich heritage of healing with plants.

# CHAPTER ONE

# A History of
# Herbal Formulary

There is no one correct way to make herbal medicine. There are, in fact, countless ways to formulate and probably as many valid methods for craftsmanship as there are herbs and herbalists. But there are still some helpful guidelines that have been handed down to us by others who have already tried our "new" ideas and either succeeded or failed. It's useful to study what people have done in the past and apply these methods to your own current situation, and also to remember that just because it works once doesn't mean it will always work. Herbs have different effects depending on where they were grown and when they were harvested, just as people respond differently to medications and herbs depending on their environment, their social interactions, and their state of mind at the moment. Flexibility is a key thing to remember and practice in the making of botanical medicine.

Since proper formulary emphasizes the best and most effective ways to combine herbs for healing, it is useful to explore the thousands of years of continuously evolving herbal principles and understanding of human anatomy. Let's briefly examine the basics of early herbal experimentation and its place within a given culture's framework of medicine.

## Prehistoric Assumptions of Healing

Throughout prerecorded history, people presumably associated healing with unseen gods and mysterious forces of nature. Sickness and healing were purely mystical experiences with no explanation and no reason. Prayer was used as the primary method of healing, and those with perceived supernatural healing abilities became known as shamans, with the term *shamanism* being applied by Western anthropologists studying the ancient religious practices of the Near East. [1]

## Shamanism

Later, some of this healing mystique rubbed off on plants, too, especially since ingesting or even touching certain plants can cause profound and immediate reactions, including sickness or death. Plants, and especially trees, were believed to possess magical qualities (such as being the portal to the gateways of death) and even to harbor powerful spirits inside them. The idea of using plants for medicine was infused with something close to a spiritual or even a religious voodoo. Healers (mostly shamans) who used plants were seen as having the special ability to transcend normal boundaries and communicate with deities most people could not. Shamans, a term eventually used to describe "magical" healers in cultures around the world, could communicate with gods, goddesses, sprites, elves, and other unseen forces and ask them to intervene, and most importantly they could

---

1    Alberts, Thomas (2015), 73–79.

communicate with the patient's own deceased ancestors, who would give guidance and power. Hence, formulary consisted mostly of spiritual communication with the divine—probably part intuition, part listening, part imagination, and part luck. Some shamans and healers were undoubtedly very skilled and began to see effects from the herbs they used; this empirical knowledge was handed down through the generations, but it was also jealously guarded. This amplified the mystique around herbs. In addition, illness was seen as retribution by the gods and punishment for deeds committed on earth. Therefore, since the cause was "supernatural," often the cure was believed to be supernatural as well, which led to many plants being labeled as magical: mistletoe and mandrake in British lore, for example.

## Supernatural Abilities of Plants

The supernatural ability of these magical plants placed them squarely in the center of certain religious beliefs. For example, the ancient Sumerian Epic of Gilgamesh tells of the superhuman king diving into the depths of the sea for the express purpose of bringing up a plant that had the power to confer immortality.[2] In the Judaic story of Genesis, the Tree of the Knowledge of Good and Evil is a magical fruit tree that confers understanding. After eating the fruit of this tree, the first woman and man are banished by God before they can eat from the Tree of Life, which would confer immortality. In both these stories it is implied that eating or tasting one of these particular plants will relieve suffering, heal the body, and sustain immortal life. Though not a "formula," it is nevertheless fascinating that the idea of plants as vehicles to long or everlasting life is an ancient concept.

## A Timeline of Theories

Mysticism did not sit well with inquiring minds who burned to know why plants behaved the way they did in the human body. By the time of

---

2    Dalley, Stephanie (2008), 39.

Hippocrates (460 BCE–c. 370 BCE), known as the "Father of Medicine," the theory of humors—using a person's temperament and coloring to diagnose illness—was well-developed and popular. Hippocrates ushered in the helpful and reasonable ideas that (a) illness is a natural occurrence (not a vindication by angry gods), (b) illness can be treated with natural (rather than supernatural) substances, and (c) the remedies can be gentle and nonviolent (rather than the violent purges used at the time). He also advanced the notion of "humors" and nearly five hundred years later, the Roman physician and philosopher Galen of Pergamon (129 CE–c. 217 CE) built on Hippocrates's idea with a strict regimen of formulas and protocols based on the theory of humors. His methods indicated an excess or deficit of one of four "liquids" in the body: black bile (melancholy), yellow bile (choleric), phlegm (phlegmatic), and blood (sanguine). Various characteristics were associated with each, including natural elements of the earth (blood with air, yellow bile with fire); physical qualities (black bile was cold and dry while an illness associated with blood was warm and moist); color; and even emotional and personality changes, including thoughtfulness and kindness. Formulary in this system was based on increasing one humor or decreasing another. The patient demonstrating hot and moist (sanguine) characteristics of illness, for instance, might be instructed to eat cold foods and cooling herbs such as chamomile or roses.

About 1,000 years after Galen, both the physician Trotula of Salerno, Italy, and the mystic nun Hildegard of Bingen, Germany, directed herbal clinics, though they used extremely different methods with varying degrees of success. Paracelsus (1493–1541) based most of his healing philosophy on the theory of humors, and even Arabic medicine, normally rational and pragmatic, succumbed in part to the idea of the humors, calling them temperaments. In 1633 John Gerard published his famous *Herball* and shortly after, in 1653, astrologically-minded Nicholas Culpeper stamped herbal medicine with his star-struck judgments of health and healing. Purging, lancing, and bleeding became favorite methods for removing excess humors, and doctors dismissed any reasonable attempts at nourishment or support.

In the 1830s, renegade herbalist Samuel Thompson challenged physician-directed medicine with assertions that it caused too much harm—often killing the patient instead of saving him, and at the turn of the nineteenth century, Quaker surgeon and inventor Joseph Lister succeeded in educating the medical profession about preventing sepsis and infection. Though popular medicine was becoming more scientifically oriented, it was still badly misshapen around the edges and quite harmful in the mainstream, with patients dying of hospital-caused infection, loss of blood, and continued ignorance of bodily functions. With the advancement of medicine, anatomy, and chemistry, modern medicine or allopathy was finally able to save lives, but it came with a price: herbal medicine, common-sense folk healing, and even the keeping of a nutritious diet were all disparaged in favor of sleek, scientific pills. Finally, in the 1960s, herbalists such as Euell Gibbons were able to reach healers with information about the intrinsic value of plants and their value as nourishing foods and gentle medicines, introducing to formulary the idea of tonics.

## Cultural Formulary

All cultures have perfected their own methods for formulary, and many formulas include not only herbs but also animal parts (such as gall bladders or paws), elemental chemicals, minerals, crystals, animal by-products (such as spider webs), and human body parts (such as hair or fingernails). Here we will deal only with healing by plants, so our formulas will be those in which herbs form the foundation of health. Some of the world's greatest healing philosophies have strong histories of using plants for this purpose and they have developed a wide following and a solid basis for efficacy.

## Ayurveda

Ayurvedic methods blossomed in India. Its process for formulary features three human traits expressed by the body as well as by thought and emotion: kapha, vata, and pitta. All of these traits are present in a person, but when they are out of balance, Ayurvedic philosophy teaches that the person will experience changes in his or her structure, function, and emotions. These traits can be measured and illness diagnosed based on the person's skin tone and color, tongue texture, activity level, mental state, and so on. Formulary is based on balancing these traits through food, massage, *materia medica* (the "collection" of medicinal plants available to the healer), drink, meditation, and exercise.

## Traditional Chinese Medicine (TCM)

TCM promotes polypharmacy, a practice that uses not just a few herbs but as many as sixty or eighty in a single formula. Traditional Chinese Medicine bases its formulary on a person's energy and "lines" of the body, assessing qi, or energy, deficient states of organs, and presence of heat or cold. In her article "Building a Formula," herbalist Chanchal Cabrera describes an interesting symbolic part of the Chinese philosophy of formulary: the primary herb in a formula symbolizes the Emperor, the secondary or adjuvant herbs symbolize Ministers of State, and warming or stimulant herbs symbolize servants.

This hierarchy of herbs by head of state easily shows which herb is "most important" or strongest, which is similar to the Western "magic bullet" approach, but it also displays the need for including supportive herbs without which the primary herb would have to work harder, and as Cabrera says, it gives a "layered" effect to the formula.[3]

---

3   Cabrera, Chanchal (2012).

# Simplers and Polypharmacy

There are countless ways to formulate medicine within a Western herbal approach, but two of the most basic ways to describe them are the simpler's method and polypharmacy.

## The Simpler's Method

One of the easiest is the simpler's method, through which the herbalist uses one herb only, assessing its various qualities and benefits for a holistic view of the patient's needs. In simple pharmacy, a single plant forms the medicine, and it can be used in a variety of ways. Simples are useful because we can clearly define a plant's action in the body and determine the pros and cons of that particular plant without having to guess which herb in a formula caused or relieved a certain symptom. Simplers have long been hailed as valuable stewards of plant medicine, and their work is of especial benefit with infants and children.

Using one herb for a variety of issues introduces a potent, singular energy to the healing experience, not to mention a greater depth of understanding of the effects of that herb. Many herbs qualify for the simpler's cabinet, especially those whose actions overlap, such as yarrow, which is at once antimicrobial, diuretic, and diaphoretic, or motherwort, which is cardiotonic, bitter, and nervine. Another is chamomile: a healer using chamomile can instruct the client to take chamomile capsules before meals for indigestion, sip hot chamomile tea before bed for insomnia, or chew bitter chamomile leaves to calm nerves.

## Polypharmacy

But what about combining herbs? What about formulary for complex blends? At a fundamental level, which herbs are best for which ailments and which are contraindicated? How much of this herb compared to that for a specific illness? Here is where formulary shines and where the handed-down knowledge of plants really gets exciting. Blending different plants together to complete a whole medicine with a variety of attributes has long been hailed as a master's level approach to herbalism, not to mention it's a lot of fun. Formulary brings together empirical knowledge of pharmacology, botany, anatomy, and—for holistic practitioners—a sense of self and intuitive integrity that is central to the healing arts.

Compound formulas, or polypharmacy, utilize many herbs in a given formula. Compound formulas sometimes include everything but the kitchen sink, though too many herbs in a formula create a burden for the body to process and expel, which can actually render a formula weak since the primary herbs are in lesser quantity.

King Mithridates VI, of Pontus and Armenia Minor from about 120–63 BCE, was a poster-child of polypharmacy. To protect himself from being poisoned, he routinely consumed small amounts of poisonous substances as a sort of homeopathic remedy. His concoction, called Mithridatum, was reported by Pliny the Elder to contain fifty-four ingredients, and he was reported to have taken daily doses of substantial poisons, but the end result, after being captured by Pompey of Rome, was that he wished to commit suicide but was unable to poison himself because his body was inured to poison. [4]

Centuries later, Galen of Pergamum experimented with this and earlier formulas (one of which contained thyme, sweet myrrh, aniseed, fennel, and parsley and was inscribed on a stone in the Kos Temple of Asclepios) and called it theriac. Galen combined fresh, dried, and fermented ingredients including snake flesh, opium, and spices mixed with honey and wine and used it both topically and internally to treat sufferers of the Antonine Plague or Plague of Galen in Rome. [5] He compounded elaborate and expensive formu-

---

4   Karaberopoulos, Demetrios, and Marianna Karamanou (May 2012). 1942–1943.

5   Ibid.

las with apparent reckless abandon, including upwards of seventy or more herbs, minerals, and crushed animal parts.

Western herbalism, on the other hand, has largely astringed its delight in multiple herbs and tends to focus on a handful, at most, in its formulary, with many herbalists including no more than six to eight herbs in a single formula. Not long ago (during the age of Samuel Thomson), this handful was condensed to exactly four. The idea was to balance an Equal-Armed Cross based on the earth's elements of earth, fire, water, and air. Proper formulas would involve each element and arm of the cross in the correct proportions.

––––––––––

Today, formulary generally takes into account the action of the herb itself, the needs of the patient (including body, mind, spirit, and social), and what herbalism has the most to offer: specific curative effects for given organs, body systems, and acute illnesses; sustainable modulating effects for chronic issues; and preventive nutritive support for long-term nourishment and balance. Western herbalists construct their formulas in various ways; Amanda McQuade Crawford calls her approach "The Triangle," since she focuses on a specific, an adjuvant, and one or more nutritive, or nourishing herbs. Her practical approach stresses the importance of understanding the energy or vibration of the patient, therapeutic priorities, the site of the primary manifestation, and the functions that need rebalancing.

Other approaches include using flavorful herbs that taste good; Oregon herbalist Cascade Anderson Geller told me that she long refused to flavor her remedies, insisting that people simply needed to take the medicines as they were. But she later changed her mind and decided to make her medicines flavorful. "I always want to improve the beauty and flavor of formulas," she says. "This was something I turned my nose up at early in my career as I felt people should take their medicines, so to speak, no matter what they tasted like. But after working with people I realized they respond better when medicines are gentler and more flavorful."[6] Many herbalists add spearmint, anise, or licorice as a corrigent, an ingredient that enhances the flavor of a formula for better tolerance.

## No Magic Bullet

Today's practice of herbalism is a rich composite of ancient medical folklore and modern scientific inquiry. We have the great benefit of thousands of years of historical use of certain herbs, as well as the clinical and scientific research of chemistry, physics, and anatomy. Combined, these sciences give us a wonderful foundation for employing plants as healing agents for the body. But I don't like to assume plants are simply "agents" for our unbridled use; rather, I teach that when used in the proper context—with respect for the natural world, with creativity, with appreciation for the pioneers who went before us, and with humility for all that we have yet to discover—plants and their medicines can become a steady and trustworthy foundation for human medicine. I advocate integrative medicine—blending herbal healing with allopathic medicine and other healing arts when needed to positively benefit the individual since every person and illness is unique and must be approached with creativity and tolerance for other modalities.

In this book, you'll be introduced to my 4-tier formula structure, which reflects some of the philosophies of these other Western methods. It's similar in that it provides primary, adjuvant (corollary or helping), and other herbs, but it tends to give greater prominence to supportive and nourishing herbs and less prominence to specific or "active" herbs, making for a balanced formula that can generally be taken with long-term sustenance in mind. Each formula begins with a general tonic or support

---

6   Bellebuono, Holly (2014).

herb for a particular organ or system of the body, followed by a "specific" herb based on the illness, followed by herbs for corollary support (or, more generally, bitters), and finally the inclusion of a "vehicle" or carrier herb, if needed, since certain herbal chemicals have been shown to congregate in and directly affect certain areas of the body, such as the uterus, the muscles, or the head. This has been a valuable approach for me as I've worked with people in a clinical setting as well as in apothecary and craftsmanship settings. *An Herbalist's Guide to Formulary* utilizes the 4-tier formula structure and offers sample protocols for a variety of issues; as always, use common sense and work in tandem with a knowledgeable health care professional in order to integrate other forms of medicine.

Over the course of the past twenty-three years, I've honed my formula-making methods and have created more than seventy original-blend products for my apothecary's retail and wholesale lines. Through trial-and-error, using intuition, working with clients, and studying within a vast heritage of herbalists from past centuries as well as those with whom I've had the pleasure of meeting and studying, I've developed successful formulas pulling from hundreds of herbs. Work with your formulas until you feel you have a practical, inspired, and most of all—effective—formula for a given illness. Part of the equation for holistic healing involves not only effective herbs and curative therapies, but also the corollary/adjunct/helpful/sidelines/sometimes-overlooked efforts of loving and caring for another person. This is the cornerstone of the healing arts.

# CHAPTER TWO

# The 4-Tier Formula Structure

Bearing all this in mind, we can begin to put together an herbal platform that will readily address many illnesses to nourish and support the person's efforts toward wellness. The formula may comprise a few different remedies given in proportion to one another; not every ingredient needs to be in the same bottle. For example, you may give certain medicines in a tea and other medicines in a topical compress, or a salve, oil, tincture, syrup, or other remedy, knowing that each remedy is part of a broader protocol for the client. You may give one tincture in the first week of therapy and change to another tincture later. The overall formula may include all of these, with you keeping in mind that all the herbs are working synergistically despite not being in the same bottle or even in the same timeframe.

We also must remember that short-term gains cannot substitute for long-term wellness. While part of our efforts must be immediate (for pain relief or symptom reduction), the holistic framework of herbalism teaches that we think long-term, that we adopt strategies that will empower the person toward wellness well into the future, and that we, as healers, engender a sense of responsibility in the person that is absent in the quick popping of a pill.

The inclusion of such an herb, so that the minimal number of herbs needed in a formula all overlap or are complementary, is called exquisite formulary. It's a graceful and harmonious blend of action, purpose, and fulfillment. In the 1990s, I worked with "the last American man" Eustace Conway at North Carolina's Turtle Island Preserve, and he told me his philosophy for efficient homesteading, which I think perfectly applies to herbal formulary. He said, "It's an economic perspective. What is the best, most streamlined use of energy? Think of it as the martial art of energy use—graceful, fine, correct choices for life." Similarly, making the most graceful and correct choices for the herbs in a formula is respectful of both the plant and the person and will result not only in better recordkeeping and observation, but ultimately in better health.

To accomplish these lasting and effective results, many herbalists develop and stick with a formula that works for them and serves as a springboard for all their formula making endeavors. I've developed a formula-making philosophy I call the 4-tier formula structure, and I generally use this as a launching pad from which I can adjust or enhance any given treatment for the most effective and nourishing remedies possible. Feel free to use this as a base for your crafting from which you can develop and pursue your own methods.

## Tier 1: The Tonic

The foundation of my formula structure is nourishment, which is tier 1, the basis of every formula. Tier 1 herbs are meant to be taken long-term to nourish, support, and sustain.

Many tier 1 herbs are precisely those sustaining herbs that we enjoy drinking as teas or infusions every day because they are delicious, mineral-rich, and "energizing" (though no tier 1 herbs contain caffeine). Examples of tier 1 herbs are lemon balm, nettle, red clover, alfalfa, ashwagandha, oatstraw and oats milky tops, gotu kola, vervain, ginkgo, red raspberry leaf, violet leaf and flower, holy basil (tulsi), and hawthorn (for a more complete list of tonic herbs, see Glossaries C and D at the end of this book). Tonics are safe, plentiful herbs that are not endangered or at-risk (see Glossary E: United Plant Savers Lists); they contain few phytochemicals (such as alkaloids) that could render them "active" or "curative" medicines, and they almost always are rich in the nutrients our bodies need, such as calcium, potassium, iron, and magnesium. Generally, tier 1 tonic herbs can be consumed safely, often as foods, and can be taken for weeks, months, or even years with positive effects.

Why would a formula not include a more power-packing remedy for tier 1 when your client is suffering from a viral, bacterial or fungal infection, or a wound or injury, or a mental or other physical illness? Because your client is not only that infection or illness. He or she is a whole person who happens to be suffering from something that is keeping him or her from attaining the greatest health potential at the moment. By addressing the client as a victim, or as the illness itself, or as a number (these are common habits in the modern system of allopathic medicine), your client loses self-respect, self-responsibility for healing, and the impetus and inspiration to get well. Instead, herbalism promotes the care of people, not diseases.

Generally, tier 1 tonic herbs are in the greatest quantity in the formula, usually twice as much as tier 2 herbs. For instance, in all the following formulas, if nettle is tier 1, it is listed as "2 parts" while peppermint, which might be the tier 2 herb, is listed as "1 part."

## Why Use Tonics?

Because tonics are the primary and largest part of a formula (especially in the 4-tier formula), it is worthwhile to more fully explore what tonic herbs and how they work. Literally, a tonic is an astringent herb that will tighten and tone tissues. But generally speaking, herbalists use a tonic (or *trophorestorative* herb) in the broad sense of an herb that will support and nourish an organ or a system of the body—not necessarily an astringent, but rather any herb that offers support, nutrients, or support for the proper, robust, and long-term function of part of the body. A tonic will help sustain a person because of its effects on an organ or system that complement all other organs and systems, since everything in the body is, of course, connected. An herb that replenishes, supports, and provides for the needs of a part of the body (or mind), and that is safe to be taken long-term, and that has few if any side effects, is a tonic—and listed as a tier 1 herb in the 4-tier formula structure.

The ultimate goal of most herbalists is to educate people in how to use tonics, because this is preventive medicine. Tier 2, 3, and 4 herbs are usually "reactive" herbs, those used when something has already gone wrong, when we are sick or injured. But tier 1 tonic herbs can be used at any time, before or after illness, and are often responsible for keeping us healthy enough that we don't need the other types of herbs. tonic herbs are our vitamin supplements and are meant to be taken daily over the course of several weeks, months, or even years. The general criteria for a tonic herb is that it:

- Is safe to use every day, long-term
- Supports and nourishes a particular organ or system of the body
- Does no harm
- Is preventive, not (necessarily) reactionary
- Enhances the efficacy of reactionary or curative herbs

I also add that a good tonic must be plentiful (not endangered or threatened), and that it provides what the body needs (i.e., it's not superfluous but is genuinely needed). Many herbalists also include the trait that a tonic is an herb with a long history of use (in any tradition). Most tonic herbs are very body-friendly, but some should not be used during certain circumstances such as hyperthyroidism (bladderwrack or kelp). But most can be enjoyed widely and with noticeable improvements for the organ or body system they support. Many people experience enhanced energy, stronger nails, teeth and hair, clearer skin, healthier libido, better metabolism, and better strength in general after using tonic herbs over a period of time.

Also, beware that some herbalists erroneously consider certain herbs such as cayenne, thyme, or garlic to be tonics for specific body systems, such as the respiratory or immune systems. I don't include these herbs here because they don't meet the definition: i.e., these are stimulants and "curative" herbs best used to work reactively as antibacterial agents against an illness for a short period of time. Cayenne, thyme, and garlic are strong herbs best used in short-term situations to reverse a given condition, not long-term as prevention, and in the formulas in this book they will feature not as tier 1 Tonics but as tier 2 specifics, tier 3 corollary, or tier 4 vehicle herbs. Stimulants are rarely used as long-term trophorestorative tonics, with the exception (in my experience) of ginger, which can be used in very small (food) doses in certain circumstances for short-term (not long-term) support. While herbs do not necessarily need to be sedative or calming, they shouldn't have stimulating action that constantly puts the body on alert or forces the body and its organs to endlessly perform. Quite the opposite—they should restore, refuel, support, and nourish.

Whereas herbal medicine differs from conventional (allopathic) medicine, so, too, do tonics differ from what most people consider herbal medicine. Allopathic medicine is usually synthetic, concentrated, fast-acting, and with side effects. It has been called "the heroic" approach since it targets symptoms and can be "warlike" in its terminology, since the doctor acts as the "hero" who saves the patient through his or her actions. Herbal medicine differs from this in that it is natural (nature-based), semi-concentrated, and much slower-acting. Herbal medicine has far fewer side effects (though side effects do exist), and it is holistic, educating, and engaging the patient in his or her own care.

Herbal tonics, while being within the realm of herbal medicine, differ again. They are natural (nature-based), not overly concentrated, very slow-acting, but much longer-lasting than either conventional or herbal specifics. They are holistic, with the responsibility for healing resting with the person (not the doctor or herbalist), and they are generally used in a preventive fashion instead of reactionary.

### Tonics (Rasayanas) in Ayurvedic Medicine

Ayurveda has a long tradition of using herbal and food tonics to replenish exhausted body systems as well, and as these philosophies and herbs differ somewhat from Western herbal medicine, it is useful to describe the basics of how Ayurvedic tonics work. Ayurvedic tonics are central to a holistic support program for individuals recuperating from illness or going through a challenging period of life. Ayurveda incorporates "rasayana" as one of its eight main branches of life study; rasayana herbs are used to nourish and replenish the body after detox and also for anyone who is in a weakened or otherwise stressed state: pregnancy, convalescent, elderly, etc. Many rasayana herbs are antioxidant and are also foods: kichari, a mixture of brown rice, mung beans, spices and ghee is one of the predominant foods eaten as a restorative tonic.[7] Grains, nuts, and seeds, milk, ghee, beans, and warming spices are also rasayana foods and tonics.

One of the biggest differences in how these two philosophies approach tonics is that whereas Western herbal medicine generally uses non-warming

---

7   McIntyre, Anne (2013), 239–243.

nutritive herbs as tonics, Ayurvedic practitioners prize the carminative and stimulating herbs and spices that stimulate vigor and metabolism: cinnamon, ginger, clove, cumin, and garlic. Many bitters are also used as tonics in Ayurveda, whereas they would normally be employed strictly as digestive aids in Western herbal medicine. The idea behind the use of spicy, bitter, and stimulating is to give that extra oomph and strengthen the entire body toward aliveness and away from sedentary "kapha" states of being. But these stimulating and sometimes spicy herbs are tempered in the overall diet with sustaining and sweet foods such as honey, maple syrup, milk, and raw sugar for a general effect of nourishment, stimulation, and true "feeding" from the inside out. Other rasayana herbs include tulsi (holy basil, or *Ocimum sanctum*, and other species), ashwagandha (*Withania somnifera*), shatavari (also spelled shatawari, *Asparagus racemosus*), amla (*Emblica officinalis*), haritaki (*Terminalia chebula*), and bala (*Sida cordifolia*).

## Difference Between Tonic and Adaptogen

In glossary A at the end of this book you'll find examples of both tonics and adaptogens with brief definitions. Though they seem quite similar on the surface, they accomplish different things in the body. In the 1960s, Russian scientists researched alternatives to *Panax ginseng*, studying a shrub native to Russia, *Eleutherococcus senticosis*, hoping to find a plant that could safely increase military performance. They created a new classification to describe its effects: adaptogen, and herbalists around the world recognized that other medicinal herbs also protect and normalize the endocrine, immune, and nervous systems, including Korean ginseng, astragalus, and echinacea. The term adaptogen now recognizes any herb that modulates the stress response and supports in a nonspecific way the vital balance between the endocrine, immune, and nervous systems.

A tonic, on the other hand, is an herb that supports, in a nonspecific way, the vital function of a particular organ or system of the body.

### Tonics and the Magic Bullet Approach

Tonics are not drugs. Tonics will work subtly, over time, often in ways that are immeasurable to those of us who like to quantify and record specific results. I have talked with many people who have given up on herbs or who remain skeptical because herbs did not work "fast enough." Now, at the beginning of the twenty-first century, people are accustomed to quick turnaround and instant gratification, and herbs have yet to catch up with them. Ancient and patient, tonic herbs are not sudden instigators; rather, they welcome gradual shifts in our bodies that lead us toward positive change. That said, I've also worked with many people who are thrilled to report substantial and lasting change due to the long-term use of tonic herbs.

Tonic herbs cannot help a person build strength and health if the person continues to indulge in poor habits such as smoking, not exercising, eating fatty, fried, or sugary foods, or embracing a negative attitude. It's best to practice an entire program of good health, using all the strategies mentioned in this book over a long period of time.

### Malnutrition

The United Nations' World Health Organization lists malnutrition as the greatest threat to public health—not influenza, lack of exercise, or even cancer. Malnutrition is inexcusable when the world produces enough food-calories to feed every person alive—and when food is routinely thrown out. Americans generated thirty-four million tons of food waste in 2010—a number only surpassed by paper and paperboard waste. Even in America, adults and children suffer severe and chronic malnutrition due to poor food choices, obesity, dysfunctional nutrient absorption, and underlying ill health. Malnutrition in children can quickly lead to poor memory and cognitive dysfunction long before physical symptoms are noticed.

Protein malnutrition, particularly in so-called underdeveloped countries—some prefer to call them under-supported countries, since (especially commercial) development is not necessarily a positive thing—is often a fatal experience. Micronutrient malnutrition can lead to severe nutrient deficiency, vomiting, and diarrhea; diarrhea, in particular, compounds the loss of micronutrients and can quickly bring death, especially for children. Malnutrition combined with social or cultural mandates (such as covering up with sunscreen in the sun or with burkas outdoors) can interfere with the body's ability to get the vitamin D it needs, which reduces its ability to absorb other nutrients such as calcium. Once the body is deficient in a mineral or vitamin, it's a short hop to deficiency in many others since their use and absorption are interdependent.

We're all aware that a deficiency in vitamin C can cause scurvy, and that once the importance of this vitamin was realized, afflicted sailors were provided with limes on voyages to prevent the disease. But nutrient deficient diseases are still common and are more plentiful than we might realize in a culture with grocery stores on every corner. In fact, many people throughout the world suffer from acute and chronic conditions that can be remedied with proper nutrition. A deficiency of iron causes anemia (which can occur after losing blood through an injury, giving birth, or experiencing menorrhagia or heavy periods). A deficiency in vitamin D can cause rickets and skeletal deformities, especially in the presence of genetic predisposition. A deficiency in iodine can cause hypothyroidism, goiter, and severe mental function impairments, with IDD (iodine deficiency disorder) causing cretinism, a dire and incurable form of mental illness.

Diets low in vitamin A can also contribute to complications of infectious diseases, such as rubella and AIDS, and undernutrition exacerbates other diseases such as measles, diarrhea, pneumonia, and malaria. A chronic lack of vitamin A can cause night blindness and vision problems, poor immune function, and growth retardation. Nearly half a million children are afflicted by blindness every year due to vitamin A deficiency, and half of these children die within a year of going blind.

Iron deficiency results in anemia, a chronic problem that afflicts an astounding 30 percent of the world's population. Anemic children suffer from cognitive disability and impairment, low birth weight, and a higher risk for infections. According to the World Health Organization, anemia contributes to 20 percent of all maternal deaths. [8]

## Tonics Are Nourishing, Nutritive Herbs

Many tonic herbs are simply nutrient-packed plants that confer their vitamins and minerals to us when we consume them, and when used long-term, especially as infusions, they can significantly impact micronutrient malnutrition. Herbs such as oatstraw, comfrey, red clover, raspberry, horsetail, and nettle are rich in calcium, iron, potassium, phosphorus, vitamins A, B, C, and more; carotenes, amino acids, chlorophyll, and fiber. Many tonic herbs are actually food herbs and can be eaten in great quantities in healthy meals: oats, nettle, dandelion leaf and root, and burdock root, to name a few. Many other edible herbs, such as chickweed, could become tonic herbs if used on a long-term basis and with the intent that they are tonics.

Tonic herbs are especially useful for three conditions:

1. Nutrient-deficit conditions (micronutrient malnutrition).

2. Specific time-constrained periods of illness, stress, or challenge, such as pregnancy, travel, school, when you want to nourish and support the body and mind for a particular event or situation.

3. Convalescence, which is the recuperation period after an illness or a stressful or strenuous time, when the body is recovering and needs nourishment and support to regain its previous level of strength and health. (See rasayanas, mentioned earlier.) During

---

8  World Health Organization (2016).

convalescence, recovery depends on the body's ability to regenerate tissues and also on the mind's ability to reconnect nerve endings, stabilize emotions, and project positively into the future. While it depends on what the person is recovering from (acute injury? respiratory illness?), common tonic herbs used during recovery periods include oatstraw (oats milky tops), slippery elm, red clover, violet leaf, self-heal, hawthorn, ginkgo, alfalfa, and nettle.

## Tier 2: The Specific

Tier 2 Specifics are the primary herb for any given condition or illness. Specifics are particular to a system of the body or directly influence the body's ability to deal with an illness, or they are capable of ridding the body of a particular disease.

Tier 2 herbs for various conditions might include goldenseal for bacterial infection, yarrow for fever, and elderflower or horseradish for sinus congestion. Tier 2 is the closest thing we'll come to in herbalism to a "magic bullet," though they're not being used that way here. When many people feel they are coming down with a cold and think, "I should take some echinacea," this is a "magic-bullet" approach; here we offer suggestions for broadening that approach to include other herbs, one of which, echinacea, may be a specific in the 4-tier formula. Instead, they're being employed to work in concert with a number of other herbs, and also they're being used with discretion in terms of quantity—often tier 2 herbs will be used in half the quantity as the tier 1 herbs, or even less, though they'll usually be in greater quantity than tier 3 or tier 4 herbs. It's also important to remember that tier 2 herbs won't be used for the length of time as tonic tier 1 herbs; for example, a person may only need horseradish (tier 2) for a few days, while they'll need the tonic benefits of nettle or elderflower (tier 1) for weeks. Be sure to adjust the formula as needed so that the specific is only being taken when it's actually needed.

# Tier 3: The Corollary

Tier 3 corollary herbs address issues that come along with an illness, or they may be bitters to support digestive health, or they may be warming herbs to support circulation. This tier is sometimes called adjuvant, supportive, corollary, or secondary. These herbs can either help the specific herb in its function (i.e., help tier 2), or they can address secondary symptoms that aren't addressed by the tier 2 specific.

For example, in the case of irritable bowel syndrome (IBS), I might employ slippery elm as the tier 3, because this herb (the soft inner bark of the slippery elm tree ground into powder) is demulcent and soothing to the gastrointestinal tract. The IBS is actually the secondary issue here while stress management is the primary issue, and soothing the gut is a secondary (though important) priority.

In an example of a topical remedy, a formula may be created for a wound that includes calendula as tier 1, yarrow as tier 2, and red clover as tier 3. All three herbs are vulnerary herbs, meaning they help heal wounds. But thinking of red clover as a tier 3 recognizes its soothing effects that are supportive, while yarrow is styptic.

Often, tier 3 herbs are warming or bitter. Warming herbs and spices "open up" a person to herbal healing, speeding blood flow and improving both digestion and circulation so that the tier 2 herbs can work effectively.

Warming herbs such as mustard, cayenne, ginger, clove, and cinnamon are especially helpful in cold or stagnant conditions, but they can also be added whenever there is mental fatigue, blockage, slow movement, or confusion.

Bitters make a wonderful tier 3 addition because they naturally stimulate the body toward active digestion, supporting a process central to daily function and indirectly supporting other tiers in the formula.

# Tier 4: The Vehicle

Finally, tier 4 herbs are the "vehicle" or "carrier," that special herb that has what herbalists call an "affinity" for a certain organ or system of the body. These herbs usher the real workers to the area of the body where they're needed, so to speak. In the case of IBS mentioned previously, I might use chamomile because it is both a nervine tonic (soothing to the emotions) and a mild bitter and carminative (soothing to the gastrointestinal tract). As a vehicle, it will "usher" other herbs, such as slippery elm, motherwort, or passionflower, to the appropriate areas of the body.

The idea of a vehicle or carrier herb may seem vague at first, but it draws from a lengthy heritage of herbalism and observation of how plants act in the body; it refers to the many instances where plant chemistry closely matches body chemistry, and certain herbs really do have a pronounced effect on certain organs or systems. For instance, feverfew and ginkgo act as vasodilator, opening the arteries and vessels and thereby increasing the blood flow to the brain; as such, these herbs could be considered tier 2 Specifics for a headache, but they could also be tier 4 vehicles when another herb is the specific. Similarly, raspberry has traditionally been considered in herbal medicine as having an "affinity" for the uterus; in formulas for pelvic inflammatory disorder or uterine cramping, raspberry could be an excellent choice as a tier 4 vehicle.

There might not be a tier 4 herb in every formula, so if there are no practical "vehicle" herbs, you may elect to leave out the tier 4 altogether, or you may choose another tier 1 or tier 3 herb to round out the formula and enhance its efficacy. In every case, the goal should be to use as few herbs as possible to achieve the greatest results. For this reason, look for those multipurpose herbs with actions that overlap—herbs that achieve many results in various body systems. Motherwort is a good example of an herb with multiple functions: it is a nervine to relieve stress, a cardiotonic to ease heart palpitations, and a bitter to stimulate proper digestion. The quantity of the tier 4 herb can be much smaller than the others; I generally list it as ½ part.

## How to Use This Book: Tiers and Parts

While each chapter discusses the anatomy, issues, and symptoms associated with the major systems of the body and suggests herbal tiers for use in formulary, the formulas are listed with "parts." This generally corresponds to the tiers and is meant to help the practitioner structure the formula in a concise and easy way, and it allows for making a small batch or a large batch. For instance, the first line of a formula generally lists "2 parts" and refers to what is normally the tier 1 tonic. The next lines generally list "1 part" and refer, in order, to tiers 2, 3, and 4.

The use of "parts" signifies that the tier 1 (herb with 2 parts) is in double the quantity as the following herbs. A formula with 2 parts nettle and 1 part chamomile is calling for double the amount of nettle in the remedy, whether it is a tea, capsule, powder, tincture, etc. It also allows the practitioner to create a small batch using teaspoons (2 parts nettle to 1 part chamomile equals 2 teaspoons nettle to 1 teaspoon chamomile) or larger measures such as cups (2 cups nettle to 1 cup chamomile). In this way, the formulas here are not recipes, but are guidelines for creating remedies based on the 4-tier formula structure. Use these guidelines as a basis for your own herbal formulas.

## Examples of Using the 4-Tier Formula Structure

Though there are no steadfast rules, the tiers in the formula begin to take shape when talking to a person and considering his or her many different needs. Let's create examples of how herbs can be placed in formulas using the 4-tier formula structure.

## Example #1: Formula for Urinary Tract Infection (UTI)

Imagine an otherwise healthy woman has been diagnosed with a urinary tract infection. We will construct a formula beginning with a nourishing tonic, which for a UTI could be dandelion or nettle (each of which performs double duty as a diuretic). A tier 2 specific for a UTI would be an antibacterial to eliminate infection: consider goldenseal, yarrow, garlic, echinacea, or Oregon grape root. Since tier 3 is for either corollary infections or issues, or it can be a bitter, we can already see that several of the tonic and specific herbs for the urinary tract are already bitters (yarrow, goldenseal, and dandelion) so these herbs could fulfill two roles in the formula. Finally, we can employ a carrier or vehicle to "transport" the other herbs directly to where they're needed: consider bearberry, dandelion, or buchu.

Using this method, we can create several effective yet very different formulae depending on what else is going on in this woman's life:

### A FORMULA FOR UTI DUE TO STRESS (AS A TEA, CAPSULE, OR TINCTURE)

› 2 parts nettle

› 1 part lemon balm

› 1 part goldenseal

› 1 part yarrow

### A FORMULA FOR UTI WITH HEART PALPITATIONS (AS A CAPSULE OR TINCTURE)

› 2 parts motherwort

› 1 part Oregon grape root

› 1 part garlic

› 1 part dandelion

## Example #2: Tonics for Cervical Health

A young woman in her late teens gets a Pap smear that shows irregular cells and indicates possible cervical dysplasia. Two formulas (one internal and one external) could be:

### A FORMULA TO SUPPORT CERVICAL HEALTH (AS A TEA TO DRINK)

› 2 parts nettle

› 2 parts raspberry

› 1 part calendula

› 1 part chaste tree berry

### A FORMULA TO SUPPORT CERVICAL HEALTH (AS A DIAPHRAGM PACK)

› 1 part pau d'arco

› 1 part calendula

## Example #3: Formula for Kidney Stones

A middle-aged man experiences kidney stones (also called gravel). Tonic herbs could include yarrow, nettle, or cleavers; Specifics could include bearberry (which reduces accumulation of uric acid, though it can change the color of the urine). Appropriate bitters include yarrow and dandelion, and carriers include bearberry, dandelion, and cornsilk.

### A FORMULA FOR KIDNEY STONES

› 2 parts dandelion

› 1 part bearberry

› 1 part yarrow

› 1 part cornsilk

## Example #4: Tonics for Enlarged Prostate

A forty-eight-year-old man experiences enlargement of the prostate gland. Tier 1 tonics could include saw palmetto, nettle root, or kelp. Tier 2 Specifics include saw palmetto, pygeum, nettle root, pumpkin seeds, green tea, and ginger. Tier 3 corollary herbs for inflammation include parsley, turmeric, and mullein (which is often thought of as strictly a respiratory herb but can be useful as a relaxing tonic in any situation). Alternatively, tier 3 bitters include gentian, dandelion, motherwort, green tea, and chamomile, while tier 4 vehicle herbs include saw palmetto.

### A FORMULA FOR ENLARGED PROSTATE

› 2 parts saw palmetto

› 1 part nettle root

› 1 part parsley

› 1 part mullein

## Example #5: Tonics for Arthritis

A middle-aged woman with lower-than-normal weight, stress, and hypertension presents with painful arthritis. We will give her two remedies: one internal as a tea, and one external that can be applied topically. The internal remedy will include tier 1 tonics and other herbs; the external remedy will not include a tier 1 tonic but will include the other tiers. In this way we are supporting her with tonic herbs for the long-term and also addressing the arthritic pain directly with a salve.

Tier 1 tonics can include nettle, dandelion leaf, and parsley, and these would be given to her as a tea while the rest of the herbs (tiers 2, 3, and 4) are given as a liniment or salve. Tier 2 Specifics can include ginger, cayenne, cinnamon, wild yam, black willow, white poplar, angelica, prickly ash, devil's claw, arnica, Jamaican dogwood, turmeric, or wintergreen (to be applied topically). Specifics for internal use for inflammation include turmeric and ginger. Corollary herbs can include ginger or prickly ash (for poor circulation), vervain or Jamaican dogwood (for insomnia especially due to pain). Bitters include dandelion leaf and motherwort while carriers include cleavers, cayenne, and prickly ash.

### A FORMULA FOR ARTHRITIS (AS A TEA TO DRINK)

› 2 parts hawthorn

› 1 part meadowsweet

› 1 part motherwort

› 1 part dandelion leaf

### A FORMULA FOR ARTHRITIS (AS A CAPSULE)

› 2 parts nettle

› 1 part turmeric

› 1 part Jamaican dogwood

› 1 part motherwort

### A FORMULA FOR ARTHRITIS (AS A TOPICAL SALVE)

› 1 part ginger

› 1 part birch

› 1 part clove

› 1 part arnica

These examples illustrate how formulas might be created for a wide variety of conditions. Be creative with your herb choices and look for ways to use edible herbs, foods, and dietary choices as supportive tonics in both the formula and dietary protocol.

Please take the basis of the information presented here and apply it in the context of your own education, adding to it, experimenting with it, and enhancing it for the greater understanding of your family, your community, and our herbal heritage at large. I encourage you to personalize this information and take what has been kneaded through history and mold it to suit your own needs. There are as many methods for making herbal medicine as there are plants, with no one perfect way, but all of our information, insights, and revelations will inform the future path of herbal healing. Also, use common sense in your approach to creating herbal formulas, understanding that specific drug–herb interactions and contraindications are beyond the scope of this book. For drug–herb interactions, collaborate with a trusted health care practitioner or knowledgeable pharmacist.

# PART TWO

# Core Body Systems

Herbal heritage contains a wealth of knowledge about the actions and uses of plants for human health. For centuries people have used plants to improve their physical and emotional states and they've carefully recorded and shared their successes. In my experience, categorizing plants by their actions is the most effective way to think about using them and to create formulas with them. Further organizing these actions by body systems makes the abundance of herbal options more easily understandable and user-friendly.

Here, we will look at three primary body systems: the digestive, cardiovascular, and respiratory systems. A complete look at every ailment possible in these systems is beyond the scope of this book, but we will create an overview of how the anatomy works and how a wide range of herbs affects that anatomy. After reviewing how each body system works and the problems most commonly associated with it, we will explore how herbal medicine can play a part in the healing of that system and specifically how to combine herbs into effective herbal formulas. Refer to the glossaries at the end of the book for more details about herbs mentioned here, as well as for suggestions about tonics for each body system.

# CHAPTER THREE

# Digestion

Digestion: for many people, this is a four-letter word. They've struggled with poor digestion, irritable bowels, and limited eating options for years. Your clients are frustrated by limiting their diet, micromanaging their meals and inevitably dealing with symptoms arising from poor digestion—including migraine headaches, gas and bloating, poor posture, and even skin disorders. Digestive disturbances usually arise from a reaction to foods, but dietary triggers are not always the cause. Many factors influence how our bodies process foods and grab needed nutrients; food allergens are an example, as are reactions to processed items in our foods, such as food colorings and artificial flavors. Additionally, emotional attitude and illness can handicap the ability to properly digest food; think of the women suffering from anorexia nervosa or bulimia, who fail to properly digest their food because of social stigmas and neuropathies that critically need professional assessment and treatment. Emotional instability and stress also play a huge part in a person's inability to properly digest food;

stress can wreak havoc not only on the stomach lining (leading to gastric ulcers when combined with the pathogen *Helicobacter pylori*), but can also lead to skin conditions including eczema and psoriasis.

Since the causes of poor digestion are numerous and much more extensive than the scope of this book will allow, we will mention a broad sampling of them but stick to how natural methods, and especially herbal medicines, can help alleviate the symptoms associated with these various and complex conditions. Combined with dietary changes, attitude adjustments, and/or specific supplements, herbal and other natural methods for relieving gastrointestinal issues are generally quite successful. You'll find here the background of many diseases and the remedies most frequently used to address those issues. Bear in mind that while many herbs will cure or treat a disease, most of the offerings here will address symptoms associated with the illness, since "curing" a disease often requires much more than a simple herbal remedy: curative actions include changing the diet, addressing the amount and types of stress in life, adjusting lifestyle choices, such as living situations and work environments, and removing toxins and allergens from the environment and the diet.

## Digestion: The Process

All mammals digest their food, a process that begins in the oral cavity and goes through all nine meters of digestive tubing in the typical human being.

From the mouth, chewed food is pushed past the esophagus and down the throat and to the stomach, where it mixes with hydrochloric acid that breaks down the food's molecular structure and kills most harmful microorganisms. Stomach acids also begin the process of breaking down proteins. From here, food goes to the small intestines, the large intestines, and is then excreted through the anus. Saliva is the first acidic compound the food encounters; then, in the stomach, the hydrochloric acid mixes with gastric juices within about two hours of eating; in the small intestines (where the food is really broken down and 95 percent of the nutrients are absorbed), bile, pancreatic juice, and intestinal enzymes, including maltase, lactase and sucrase, act on what used to be your spaghetti dinner. From here, the large intestine (also called the gut) can readily absorb the remaining nutrients and funnel them into the bloodstream. The liver is an organ that deserves an entire book of its own; it is a vital participant in digestion, maintaining protein synthesis, metabolism, hormone production, glycogen storage, and the decomposition and elimination of spent hormones and red blood cells. Proper liver function is essential for red blood cell production, emulsifying fats, and maintaining smooth hormonal activity. Without a properly functioning digestive system, our bodies could not access the vitamins, minerals, proteins, enzymes, fiber, chlorophyll, and sugars that are available to us in our foods.

Following are protocols for general digestive health, and following *those* are a variety of digestive disorders and natural methods for addressing them.

## General Protocols

Protocols for healthy digestion often reflect protocols for healthy eating in general, with just a few exceptions that take into consideration a person's proclivity for gas, indigestion, acid reflux, or other symptoms. Include these as appropriate within the context of any herbal assessment.

### Protocol #1

Eat less. This is the core of any program for dieting to lose weight, but it's also helpful to address a digestive disorder. Instead of big meals, eat several small meals or snack throughout the day. Distending the stomach is easy to do and hard to reverse, and the feeling of fullness contributes to lethargy, mental fogginess, and distress.

## Protocol #2

Eat more fiber. Unless a client suffers from diverticulitis, in which tiny pouches form on the inside of the large intestine and become inflamed, encourage the addition of fiber in his or her diet. Today's American diet of refined wheat flours, white breads, white rice, and frozen dinners with squashy vegetables preserved with sodium is a healthy eater's nightmare. Refining flours removes not only the vitamin-rich germ, but also strips the grain of its natural fiber. Your gut depends on fiber to push the waste products through and to expel them properly. Improper amounts of fiber in the diet can lead to diarrhea or constipation. Nutrients are not absorbed and toxins are not expelled properly. Good sources of fiber include fresh, raw foods and whole grains, as well as legumes of all kinds (especially lentils and black beans), broccoli, raw apples, oats, barley, pumpkin, and garden squashes. Surprisingly, avocado tops the list of fiber-dense foods, providing 11 grams of fiber per medium avocado (compared to 4 grams of fiber per medium raw apple). Also, dried fruits such as figs, apricots, and dates are packed with fiber. Snack on these, or chop them up and include them in your breakfast cereal, whole grain bread recipes, green salads (their sweet flavors contrast nicely with tart vinegars), and in Indian and Thai dishes. Encourage clients to eat whole grain breads, rice, and even pastas and pastries—and to serve these with salsa, shredded cheese, baked sweet potatoes with the skins on, chopped avocado, a small amount of pork, turkey or beef, if desired, and a liberal sprinkling of Mexican oregano, cumin, chili powder, and paprika—for a total of a 1-cup meal.

## Protocol # 3

Remove gas-forming foods from the diet if gas and bloating are a cause of concern. Many people experience gas (flatulence), bloating, burping, indigestion, and other symptoms that indicate a food sensitivity. Cabbage (or any member of the *Brassica* family), peanuts, orange juice, and beans are common causes, as is sugar in any form. Carbonated beverages are a common gas-causer, of course, and these include sodas, beer, and carbonated water. Other gas-forming foods include fried foods, rich dairy-based foods, and (unhelpfully) most of our best fiber-rich foods. Experiment with the fiber foods to determine if any need to be removed because of gas production, but don't eliminate them altogether—fiber is essential for proper digestion. Pseudo foods are marketed as ingredients but are actually not natural and often cause gas. Avoid high fructose corn syrup, hydrogenated oils, partially hydrogenated oils, and monosodium glutamate. Stomach aches, nausea, headaches, skin rashes, blurry vision, and heart palpitations are symptoms of a possible food allergy that warrants immediate attention and possibly a trip to the emergency room. Common allergens include peanuts, wheat, dairy, strawberries, nuts of all kinds, seafood (especially shrimp and other shellfish), and eggs. These ingredients can appear in a number of seemingly innocent places. For instance, peanuts and peanut residue can appear in cookies, puddings, gravies, sauces, and even hot sauce and hot chocolate. Ethnic foods often contain peanuts—even egg rolls and salsa.

## Protocol #4

Think immune-building. Strengthen both the digestive and immune systems by eating foods that stimulate positive immune response or that kill unwanted bacteria, viral infections, fungal infections, and parasites. Some foods empower the immune responses of the body to attack and remove these from the digestive tract and the blood. Immune building foods and herbs include garlic, ginger, hot spices, and spicy foods, lemon, limes, lemongrass, cinnamon, vitamin C–rich foods, such as rose hips, and colorful fruits and vegetables, such as peppers, chard, and kale. Avoid foods that do not actively build your immune system: sugar, yeast, pseudo-foods, such as hydrogenated oils, and refined or processed foods have no place in an immune-supportive diet. Practice an immune supportive diet even if you're not sick, creating a proactive diet and food habit.

## Protocols for Specific Digestive Issues

Following are protocols with guidance for addressing basic complaints.

### Liver Health (Including Hepatitis and Jaundice)

Liver illness can be caused by a wide range of forces often outside our control. Stress on the liver can cause this important organ to fail in its vital functions, leading to symptoms in other areas of the body, such as the skin. We often fail to connect skin issues, or digestive issues, with liver stress, but if the liver can't perform its job of excreting toxins through the kidneys, it will underperform, and other waste-removing organs, such as the skin, will compensate. This often results in eczema or psoriasis. Degenerative liver failure also presents with digestive symptoms.

Liver degenerative diseases such as cirrhosis primarily affect smokers, drinkers, those suffering with hepatitis, and those working in environmentally poor conditions (industries, factories, road crews, paint stores, etc.). Women with extreme hormonal imbalances must take extra good care of their livers since one of the functions of this essential organ is to remove excess metabolic waste (i.e., spent hormones) from the bloodstream. Those with a poor diet (excess sugars, refined carbohydrates) are taxing their livers unnecessarily with an onslaught of metabolic and food wastes.

Supporting liver health will result in stronger digestion, healthier skin, clearer thinking, and balanced hormones. Eat fiber-rich foods throughout the day but especially at night, so the digestive tract can process the food during sleep and expel the waste in the morning; eat bitters in the morning and early afternoon; nap during the afternoon if stress is a contributing factor to liver illness.

Tier 1 tonics for liver illnesses are nourishing; they are sustaining herbs that offer long-term wellness regardless of the symptoms and are free from damaging alkaloids that will further tax the liver. Tonics can address stress and nervous system or they can be hepatoprotective, directly supporting liver tissue regenesis. Tier 1 tonics include dandelion root, nettle, and lemon verbena (which is considered a specific in European Western herbalism).

Tier 2 Specifics include:

- **milk thistle** (*Silybum marianum*): the seed has traditionally been used for hepatitis and cirrhosis; modern research supports its use in counteracting poisons and toxins, reducing alcohol damage, and protecting against viral toxins.[9]

- **licorice** (*Glycyrrhiza glabra*): effective against viral infection of the liver (including hepatitis and herpes). Contraindicated in hypertension.

- **schisandra** (*Schisandra chinensis*): called wu wei zi in Chinese (five flavored fruit), this tart/tangy/bitter/astringent berry of the schisandra vine has been the subject of extensive research in Russia and more recently in Europe. Showing a wide diversity of actions, this herb is considered an adaptogen and immune modulator. Its high lignan content also demonstrates hepatoprotective actions against viral infection and metal toxicity.[10][11]

- **bupleurum** (*Bupleurum falcatum*): high in saponins, bupleurum has been used traditionally in Japanese and Chinese herbalism to support immunity and reduce pain and inflammation in the thoracic and abdominal cavities. Useful for chronic hepatitis.[12]

---

9   Hoffmann (2000).

10  Panossian and Wikman (2008).

11  Winston (2013).

12  Hoffmann (1996).

- **burdock root** (*Arctium lappa*): a weed in North America and a food in the Orient, burdock produces wide, scalloped leaves and clinging seeds. Its root penetrates deeply and is used as a food and a medicine; known as a hepatic herb, burdock root is a tier 1 tonic or tier 2 specific when supporting the liver.

- **echinacea** (*Echinacea* spp.): its polysaccharides are renowned for stimulating the immune system, specifically for viral, bacterial and fungal infections such as candida and even on cancer cells. It activates macrophage response in many systems of the body and is directly useful in the digestive system; useful as a tier 3 corollary in hepatic conditions.

Tier 3 corollary herbs address headache, constipation, diarrhea, and/or suppressed immunity. Consider chamomile, turmeric, motherwort, as well as:

- **cleavers** (*Gallium aparine*): a lymph system tonic, cleavers (also spelled clivers) supports the movement of fluids in the body and can be considered anywhere there is stagnation or lack of drainage. Useful for urinary infection, skin eruptions, and liver health.

Tier 4 vehicle herbs include dandelion root and milk thistle.

### *Liver Health Formulas*
#### A FORMULA FOR HEPATITIS (AS A TINCTURE OR CAPSULE)

> › 2 parts echinacea
>
> › 1 part milk thistle
>
> › 1 part gentian or rue
>
> › 1 part dandelion leaf
>
> › 1 part dandelion root

### A Formula for Jaundice (in adults) (as a tea, tincture or capsule)

› 2 parts dandelion root

› 2 parts dandelion leaf

› 1 part prickly ash

› 1 part lemon verbena

› 1 part milk thistle

### A Formula for Liver Support

› 2 parts dandelion leaf

› 1 part milk thistle

› 1 part burdock root

› 1 part cleavers

## Indigestion and Irritable Bowel Syndrome

Irritable Bowel Syndrome consists of various symptoms that have some definite cause, but the cause is (as yet) unknown and (usually) unlooked for. Doctors seldom pursue the cause and instead prescribe over-the-counter medications to soothe the lining of the stomach or digestive tract, leaving the diet and the cause of the symptoms up to the patient to figure out.

Stress and digestion go hand in hand; stress can impact how our bodies absorb food, and indigestion can cause pain and stress. Each worsens the other. Working to remove stress from daily life (and learning how to deal effectively with stress beyond our control) is essential and is fully half the protocol for dealing with indigestion or IBS; the other half is diet.

General indigestion should be addressed with basic, common sense methods such as eliminating foods individually from the diet, reducing the quantity of food eaten, and keeping a record of foods and drinks ingested. Adequate sleep, stress reduction, and positive outlook all have a healing impact on indigestion.

Many people find benefit in a diet reduction and recording process. All at once, remove all non-essential foods from the diet. This includes crackers, chips, junk food, coffee, alcohol, sweets, snacks, salad dressing, gravy, and other foods and beverages not truly needed for proper metabolism and nutrients. Keep them out of the diet for one full week, living solely on those essential foods such as rice, vegetables, and low-sugar fruits (such as apples and pears). Carefully record everything eaten—even the seasonings. After one week, slowly add one food or seasoning back into the diet and record any symptoms, including obvious digestive symptoms as well as not-so-obvious concerns such as headache, mood swings, swelling, fatigue, and poor concentration. (For nursing infants with colic symptoms, the mother should perform these changes in her diet.)

Carminative herbs can be very helpful here; these are the aromatic herbs such as fennel, dill, sage, lemon verbena, and chamomile that help smooth the digestive process. Demulcent herbs can also be effective here, especially licorice, oats milky tops, and slippery elm.

### Indigestion and Irritable Bowel Syndrome Formulas
#### A FORMULA FOR INDIGESTION/IRRITABLE BOWEL SYNDROME

› 2 parts nettle

› 2 parts oatstraw

› 1 part lemon balm

› 1 part spearmint

### Crohn's Disease and Inflammatory Bowel Disease

Crohn's disease and inflammatory bowel disease (IBD) usually affect the intestines but may be present anywhere in the gastrointestinal area, including the rectum or the mouth. It is generally categorized as an autoimmune disease, meaning it appears to be the body's response to a perceived antagonist or allergen. The body's immune system overreacts by swelling, causing painful inflammation and poor nutrient absorption due to thick-ened intestinal wall lining. The most common symptoms include gastric and pelvic cramping, diarrhea, loss of appetite, fever, fatigue, and some-times pain with passing stools.

Generally, people between the ages of fifteen and thirty-five are those who present with Crohn's disease and IBD, suggesting a variety of theories (including dietary, genetics, and allergy—as opposed to aging and tissue breakdown). Often genetics are implicated, as those with a family history of Crohn's are more likely to present, as well as people with Jewish heritage. Smokers are at a higher risk of presenting with IBD. Stress may also be a key factor, though it tends to be neglected in most conventional literature. Many doctors prescribe antibiotics, salicylates, and even corticosteroids to treat Crohn's, but there are also proven (though not easy) dietary guidelines and herbs that can ease symptoms and make life more pleasant.

Since Crohn's can affect a wide range of locations in the body, proper diagnosis and work with a health care practitioner are essential for balanced treatment. Symptoms can show up in the stomach, the rectum, on the anus, in the mouth, on the skin, and even on the eyes. Joint pain is common, as is fever and fatigue. Because these symptoms closely mirror Lyme disease, mononucleosis, and influenza, it is critical to get an accurate diagnosis.

The above protocols for smaller meals, healthy foods, and avoidance of dairy and fatty foods are useful here, as is reducing fiber if there is pain in passing stools. The swollen tubing of the digestive system may hamper proper movement of high-fiber foods, so minimizing the fiber in this case is justified. Also avoid foods that cause gas, as bloating and cramping are already common symptoms of this disease, as well as gluten-containing foods such as wheat breads.

Crohn's sufferers must avoid inflammation-causing foods, such as dairy, wheat, eggs, nuts, spicy foods, fried foods, and fatty foods. Avoid refined sugars, but eat plenty of raw foods and foods high in beta carotene, includ-ing carrots, pumpkin, and sweet potatoes (yams). Limit deadly nightshade foods such as tomatoes, eggplants, and potatoes. And food additives contribute to inflammatory conditions; avoid aspartame, monosodium glutamate (MSG), trans-fats, carrageenan (often found in cheeses and non-dairy milk substitutes), waxes such as carnauba and candelilla wax, and emulsifiers and thickeners.

In addition to fennel, fenugreek, dill, and chamomile, other tier 2 Specifics include anti-inflammatories and carmatives:

- **wild yam** (*Dioscorea villosa*): a key anti-inflammatory, wild yam directly affects the pelvic region and is useful for abdominal cramping, gas, and uterine cramping.

- **lemon balm** (*Melissa officinalis*): high in the volatile oils that make this a prime carminative and also nervine tonic, lemon balm is useful for both the anxiety that Crohn's can cause as well as the physical symptoms of gas, bloating, and constipation.

- **lemon verbena** (*Aloysia citrodora*): considered a hepatic (liver tonic) in Western herbal medicine.

- **turmeric** (*Curcuma longa*): often used for arthritis and rheumatic inflammation but it can contribute as a remedy for bowel inflammation.

- **ginger root** (*Zingiber officinale*): As a warming herb, ginger addresses a variety of problems, especially gas and sluggish digestion. I suggest using fresh ginger in cooking and powdered ginger in as many places as possible (honey, hot teas, grains, beans, etc.).

Tier 3 corollary herbs include bitters, antispasmodics and demulcents:

- **chamomile** (*Matricaria recutita*): a mild bitter, chamomile is also a nervine and helps reduce spasms and indigestion caused by anxiety.

- **motherwort** (*Leonurus cardiaca*): a good overlap herb, motherwort addresses three body systems: digestion, cardiovascular, and nervous. Can be used as tier 1, tier 2 or tier 3 for both Crohn's and IBD. Short-term use is best; take as a capsule or tincture for up to 4 weeks.

- **cramp bark** (*Viburnum opulus*): useful for relieving muscle cramps; calms uterine and digestive cramps.

- **aloe vera** (*Aloe vera*): an excellent demulcent, aloe calms, cools and soothes cases of severe swelling or constipation. The juice is available at health food stores and can be consumed orally or dabbed on topically to soothe anal fissures and bleeding sores. Other demulcent (soothing) herbs that can be taken as thick teas include marshmallow root, plantain leaf, slippery elm powder, and arrowroot.

- **Boswellia** (*Boswellia* spp.): used in Ayurvedic methods, boswellia is mildly detoxifying and anti-inflammatory. Boswellic acids are specified in the treatment of Crohn's disease and can be taken as tablets or capsules, available at most health food stores.

- **cat's claw** (*Uncaria guianensis, U. tomentosa*): a tropical vine found throughout South America and Asia, cat's claw has been used by South American Indian cultures for centuries and is now undergoing trials to gauge its efficacy as an anti-inflammatory. Scientists believe cat's claw may suppress tumor necrosis factor (TNF), making it a possible remedy for tumors and cancers. This anti-TNF activity is anti-inflammatory in the bowels, as well, making cat's claw a potential remedy for Crohn's disease.[13]

---

13   Holly Phaneuf (2005).

Topically, applications of witch hazel, goldenseal, and plantain are useful for rectal bleeding and painful sores on the anus. Apply these with a cotton ball, or brew them into a tea and use a toilet or "sitz bath" tray (available at pharmacies), or infuse the herbs in oil and melt with beeswax to make a salve that is applied topically.

## Crohn's Disease and Inflammatory Bowel Disease Formulas

### A FORMULA FOR CROHN'S DISEASE WITH CRAMPS (AS A TEA, TINCTURE, OR CAPSULE)

› 2 parts lemon verbena

› 1 part wild yam

› 1 part cramp bark

› 1 part boswellia

### A FORMULA FOR CROHN'S DISEASE WITH ANAL FISSURES (AS A TEA, TINCTURE, OR CAPSULE)

› 2 parts chamomile

› 1 part aloe vera

› 1 part fennel

› 1 part slippery elm

## Gastric and Peptic Ulcers

Ulcerations in the soft tissues of the gastrointestinal tract deserve attention and care; left alone, ulcers often heal themselves, but they can also get worse and cause tears and holes in the lining of the stomach or the duodenum. Ulcers appear to have two primary causes: stress and depression, which can contribute to an overproduction of stomach acids, and a pathogen called *Helicobacter pylori*, a bacterial infection present in patients with chronic gastritis and gastric ulcers, is a primary culprit. Scientists believe this bacteria, which may be a common resident in most healthy people's bodies, is linked to duodenal ulcers and stomach cancer. Ulcers may also result from radiation therapy.

Symptoms of *H. pylori* infection include nausea and stomach pain, with severe cases showing bloating and vomiting. Other symptoms include a burning sensation in the abdomen, pain after eating, pain that may be relieved by drinking milk or milk products, belching, and poor appetite. Though physician-directed tests (including endoscopy and urease tests) are needed to accurately determine the presence of this pathogen, mild cases of infection and ulceration can be dealt with using herbs and diet. (NOTE: cholecystitis, or gall bladder disease, can present the following symptoms: jaundice, dark urine, rapid heartbeat, fever, chills, nausea, and specifically pain in the upper right abdomen. Other emergency issues present with symptoms such as sudden and severe sharp pain in the abdomen, vomiting blood or a substance resembling coffee grounds, and bloody stools. Seek immediate medical attention if you or your client demonstrates these symptoms.)

Stomach ulcers (gastric ulcers) appear in the mucosal lining of the stomach and often result from taking certain pharmaceutical drugs, such as aspirin or NSAIDS (non-steroidal anti-inflammatory drugs, such as ibuprofen). They are worsened with alcohol consumption.

Common solutions for the symptoms of ulcers include over-the-counter medications such as Pepto Bismal, or milk of magnesia, which is magnesium hydroxide. Antacids (such as Tums) are concentrations of calcium carbonate with other minerals and electrolytes. Magnesium hydroxide itself, because of its magnesium salts, sodium, and potassium, is considered an electrolyte, which may be part of its efficacy. Since it is also a strong laxative, Maalox is used as an antacid instead. Additionally, sodium bicarbonate (Alka-Seltzer) is a common conventional-medicine remedy for ulcers.

We are at an advantage because we have herbs that are digestively soothing (antacid), demulcent, and antibacterial. Tier 2 Specifics include:

- **licorice** (*Glycyrrhiza glabra*): licorice has long been a traditional remedy for easing stomach upsets, and is appreciated by both the herbal and allopathic communities for relief of peptic and gastric ulcers. Licorice can be taken in many forms: as a tablet, lozenge, capsule, tincture, tea, and chewing the chopped root. Many herbalists will warn to consume only DGL, which is de-glycyrrhizinated licorice, but this is not always necessary. If you or your client suffers from insufficient adrenal function, use DGL, as the triterpene glycyrrhizin can affect an unhealthy adrenal cortex. Avoid licorice in clients with high blood pressure.

- **mastic** (*Pistacia lentiscus*): traditionally used to lower high blood pressure, mastic can relieve peptic ulcers. This resinous material has many applications, though its long-term effects in humans have not been the subject of many scientific studies. For peptic or gastric ulcer, try mastic capsules for up to four weeks, but avoid in clients with nut allergies.

- **spearmint** (*Mentha spicata*): symptomatic relief for pain and discomfort of duodenal, peptic, and gastric ulcers. Full of volatile (essential) oils, mints aid in digestive function, reduce gaseous symptoms, and even lift the spirits by acting as nervine tonics. Spearmint teas or tinctures can reduce complaints associated with ulcers, whether caused by stress, NSAIDs, or *Helicobacter pylori*.

- **cranberry** (*Vaccinium macrocarpon*): may inhibit the growth of *Helicobacter pylori* in the stomach, giving reason to assume that this fruit can be used medicinally to treat gastric and peptic ulcers. Take 400 milligrams. twice daily or drink the fresh juice if renal or bladder infection is also a concern.

For *H. pylori* induced ulcers (and also for infection of *Candida albicans*), include probiotics, such as yogurts and supplements containing concentrated amounts of *Lactobacillus* and *Bifidobacterium,* in the diet. Eat fresh, unsweetened yogurt several times daily. Avoid alcohol, NSAIDS, fried foods, and trans fats such as hydrogenated oils.

### Gastric and Peptic Ulcers Formulas
#### A FORMULA FOR GASTRIC ULCER WITH NAUSEA (AS A TEA, TINCTURE, OR CAPSULE)

> › 2 parts slippery elm
> › 2 parts skullcap
> › 1 part echinacea
> › 1 part chamomile

#### A FORMULA FOR GASTRIC ULCER WITH INFLAMMATION (AS A TEA, TINCTURE, OR CAPSULE)

> › 2 parts licorice
> › 1 part passionflower
> › 1 part cranberry
> › 1 part slippery elm

### Diverticulitis

Diverticulitis is the inflammation of the diverticuli, the small sacs that line the mucosa of the colon. While the presence of sacs is common, their swelling is not, and it will impede the passage of matter through the colon, irritate the colon lining, and cause pain, tenderness, and even fever. Since movement of matter is affected, constipation and diarrhea often result, one after the other. Causes include stress, lack of physical activity, and especially a low-fiber-highly-refined diet typical of Western countries. However, simply increasing fiber will not necessarily cure the problem—especially in the beginning of treatment, since the person is not accustomed to high fiber and its sudden appearance can trigger painful blockages in the digestive system. Generally, diverticulitis affects the aging population, as poorer digestive ability and movement occurs as people age.

Gradually increasing the amount of fiber in the diet is key, since a diet of highly refined foods causes diverticuli to swell. Begin not with over-the-counter fiber powders, but instead with foods high in soluble fiber, such as strawberries, celery, oats, lentils, apples, dried peas and beans, and psyllium or plantain seeds, a natural treat that can be enjoyed on most foods. After these gel forming–soluble fibers have been gradually introduced and accepted by the digestive system, begin introducing insoluble fibers that add bulk to the diet and help prevent constipation, such as wheat bran, corn bran, nuts, barley, green beans, dark leafy vegetables, raisins, brown rice, bulgur, and root vegetables with their skins.

Bacterial infection is a big risk with diverticulitis, since blockages naturally impede the movement of fecal matter. Antibiotics are routinely given to prevent or reverse bacterial infections, but antibiotics will not be the first method a holistic practitioner jumps to in cases of diverticulitis. Anti-inflammatory herbs, carminative herbs, antibacterial herbs, a high-fiber diet (increasing gradually), and a program of increasing physical activity and exercise support diverticulitis. The best tier 2 Specifics are:

- **wild yam** (*Dioscorea villosa)* has a direct action on the pelvic region, reducing inflammation in the uterus and digestive system.

- **chamomile** (*Matricaria recutita*): carminative, antispasmodic, and nervine, chamomile's mild bitter qualities make it ideal for easing gas and the spasms associated with diverticulitis.

Tier 3 corollary herbs are antispasmodic and nervine:

- **valerian** (*Valeriana officinalis*): traditionally used as a sedative, a spasmolytic, and a nervine, this overlap herb addresses multiple symptoms for the person suffering diverticulitis, Crohn's, IBD, and other digestive complaints, especially those that are chronic and lead to irritability or insomnia.

Carminative herbs such as chamomile, spearmint, dill, and fennel are also useful, since they stimulate proper digestion and act as nervine tonics (consider also lemon balm, skullcap, passionflower, if stress is high). If infection is present, consider mild antimicrobials such as yarrow (also a bitter and an astringent, so use it carefully), calendula, or peppermint. Ginger can be helpful if there is flatulence, or constipation.

### Diverticulitis Formulas
#### A FORMULA FOR DIVERTICULITIS WITH GAS (AS A TEA, TINCTURE, OR CAPSULE)
› 2 parts lemon balm

› 1 part wild yam

› 1 part spearmint

› ½ part ginger

# Symptoms Indicating Diseases

The previous section dealt with specific diseases of the gastrointestinal tract. This section introduces symptoms that are not diseases but indicators of a problem that needs addressing. It is vitally important to seek medical attention if normal herbal therapy does not ease the symptom in a reasonable period of time, since these symptoms can indicate more serious problems.

### Gas and Bloating

Flatulence, or gas, is a painful and often embarrassing symptom that everyone experiences at some time or other. In infants, colic (gas and cramping) is generally assumed to be a condition of food intolerance, where the baby's digestive system can't readily digest a nutrient coming through the mother's breast milk. Often, if the mother changes her diet, the problem disappears (cabbage, garlic, onions, and broccoli are common triggers). Mother's can drink teas with carminative herbs such as anise, fennel, spearmint, or chamomile; the chemical components will be absorbed into the milk and passed on to the baby. Baby's colic may also be caused by blockages or improper tissue development; if the baby's symptoms do not improve or seem severe, consult a pediatrician.

Gas and bloating in children and adults can have a wide range of causes, including stress, anxiety, fear, drug use (prescription or otherwise), physical obstructions (seek emergency help immediately!), dietary intolerance or allergy, or lack of physical exercise and body movement. Carminative herbs are those that contain volatile oils that stimulate bile and gastric juice production and keep gas under control; these are the tier 2 herbs in most any formula for gas. Thanks to their essential oils, carminatives taste good and make pleasant teas. Consider chamomile, spearmint, peppermint, pennyroyal*, fennel, fenugreek, anise, licorice, ginger, dill, cinnamon*, cardamom, sage, thyme, lemon balm, hops, angelica, and wintergreen*. (* avoid in pregnancy)

Many carminative herbs are also anti-spasmodic, which can be helpful in reducing gas and cramping. Ginger and oregano are key here. Wild yam, valerian, and cramp bark are anti-inflammatory and reduce spasms in the gut.

### Gas and Bloating Formulas
#### A FORMULA FOR FOOD-TRIGGERED GAS

> › 2 parts chamomile

> › 1 part fennel

> › 1 part spearmint

### A Formula for Anxiety-Triggered Gas

> › 2 parts chamomile
>
> › 1 part lemon balm
>
> › ½ part ginger

### A Formula for Pre-Menstrual Gas and Bloating

> › 2 parts wild yam
>
> › 1 part chamomile
>
> › 1 part dandelion
>
> › 1 part fenugreek

## Diarrhea

A symptom and not a disease, diarrhea is the body's method of removing pathogens including bacterial and viral irritants. Diarrhea's primary threat is the loss of water and, as a result, the loss of electrolytes. Children and the elderly are the most at-risk, while travelers often experience diarrhea as a result of consuming foreign pathogens through water consumption.

Regardless of the cause, herbal treatment involves astringent herbs. Mild astringent herbs are often sufficient for stabilizing the person enough so that fluids and electrolytes can be taken by mouth without loss.

### Mild astringents

> › chamomile (*Matricaria recutita*)
>
> › raspberry leaf (*Rubus idaeus*)
>
> › plantain leaves (*Plantago major* or *P. lanceolata*)
>
> › spearmint leaves (*Mentha spicata*)
>
> › fennel seed (*Foeniculum vulgare*)
>
> › cranesbill (*Geranium maculatum*)

## Medium Astringents

> yarrow (*Achillea millefolium*)

> blackberry bark or root (*Rubus villosus*)

> shepherd's purse (*Capsella bursa-pastoris*)

> witch hazel leaves and twigs (*Hamamelis virginiana*)

> sage (*Salvia* spp.)

## Strong Astringents

> oak bark and galls (*Quercus* spp.)

> black catechu leaves (*Acacia catechu*)

Strong astringents should be used with caution and only in extreme situations.

Dysentery is an acute infection of the bowels after contamination with virulent pathogens via the mouth; called the Flux in antiquity, it results in severe diarrhea which is frequent, bloody, marked by spasms, and lasts for several days. The Flux has, throughout history, been a primary killer, taking the lives of men, women, children, travelers, and soldiers. More than 80,000 Union soldiers died of dysentery during the four years of America's Civil War. Dysentery requires immediate medical attention and treatment to kill the parasite and replace lost electrolytes.

## *Diarrhea Formulas*
### A Formula for Diarrhea (as a tea)

> 2 parts raspberry leaf

> 1 part sage

> 1 part yarrow

> 1 part chamomile

### ANOTHER FORMULA FOR DIARRHEA (AS A TEA)

› 2 parts sage

› 1 part raspberry leaf

› 1 part catnip

› 1 part oatstraw

## *Constipation*

Another symptom (not a disease itself), constipation is the loss of movement in the bowels, resulting in blockages, cramps, bloating, and sometimes fever. Bacterial infection is also a common side effect and can be dealt with using antibacterial herbs.

Constipation has a wide range of causes: stress can cause constipation, since we naturally tend to "tighten" when we are anxious or worried. Other causes include dehydration, poor nutrition, lack of probiotics, fear (question whether the person is uncomfortable in his/her surroundings or is experiencing a threat), diverticulitis, physical obstruction (seek immediate emergency attention), or too much fiber.

Constipation can often be regulated with diet and with herbs. If the person is normally experiencing bouts of constipation without fever or other problems, the use of herbs may be beneficial in "reprogramming" the bowels and gastric organs to perform normally.

Demulcent herbs are useful here: slippery elm, oats milky tops, and mallow. Anti-spasmodic herbs include cramp bark, ginger, and turmeric. "Wet" herbs that are slick and juicy and speed the flow of fluids through the digestive system can also help with constipation: nettle, dandelion, and aloe vera.

*Constipation Formulas*

### A Formula for Constipation (as a tea)

> › 2 parts nettle

> › 1 part plantain

> › 1 part aloe vera

> › ½ part ginger

Nourishing the digestive system and relieving symptoms of digestive disorders can be accomplished using herbs, common sense, compassion, and proper diet. Don't be afraid to try new herbs, or in new combinations, as each person is different, has unique needs, and responds to herbal medicines differently.

CHAPTER FOUR

# Cardiovascular

The heart is arguably one of the most fascinating organs of the mammalian body; in the human being, the heart begins its formation, as early as twenty-one days after conception, in the shape of a simple tube; this tube folds in on itself and forms four chambers thirty-four days after conception. Barely a month old, the embryo now has a fully functioning beating heart, though the circulatory and vascular systems will take many more months to complete their amazing development.

The heart is comprised of myocardial muscle, one of the three types of muscle cells (the other two are smooth and skeletal muscle). It is an organ located behind the ribs, just to the left of the sternum, that is divided into four chambers: the right and left atrium, and the right and left ventricle. The right atrium brings blood from the body that has traversed the circulatory system and distributed its oxygen; this blood is pumped through the tricuspid valve into the right ventricle, which shunts the blood through the pulmonary valve, into the pulmonary artery, and straight into the lungs. After collecting fresh new oxygen, the blood is pumped by the ventricle through the pulmonary veins up to the left atrium and then into the left ventricle; from here, the blood courses through the aortic valve to the aorta and on to the rest of the body. This entire process is based on electrical impulses.

With the average adult's heart rate between seventy and eighty beats per minute (about one hundred thousand times per day), it takes approximately one minute for blood to make its circulation throughout the entire body. During strenuous exertion, an adult's blood may complete its circulation of the body in as little as twenty seconds, a remarkable feat considering it has roughly one hundred thousand miles of veins and arteries to travel—almost half the distance from the Earth to the moon.

Veins carry blood to the heart to re-oxygenate, while arteries carry oxygenated blood to other parts of the body. Arteries require the direct pumping action of the heart to move blood because they depend on the pressure caused by the heart's pumping action and the restriction of the size of the artery; veins, on the other hand, use one-way valves that are controlled by the contraction of muscles. For this reason, arteriolosclerosis and atherosclerosis are so dangerous, because the more compacted an artery is with cholesterol-based plaque, the less efficient its pumping action and the greater the pressure is exerted on the tissues of the artery.

## General Protocols for the Heart

According to the World Health Organization, more people die globally from cardiovascular disease (including coronary heart disease and stroke) than from any other cause. [14] The WHO lists unhealthy diet, physical inactivity, and tobacco use as top causes of cardiovascular disease. Obesity is known to severely complicate the workings of the heart and the circulatory

---

14   Cardiovascular Diseases (2016).

system; the pressure on the body's cavities and vessels is great, not to mention the excessive amounts of cholesterol-based plaque that form on vessels from a poor diet. If the obesity is caused by hormonal or glandular issues, then the cardiac muscle and system is already compromised.

Smoking is often hailed as the number one cause of heart disease, but why? What is it about tobacco that makes it such a detriment to heart health? Tobacco smoke directly reduces blood circulation and constricts blood vessels; this raises blood pressure and deprives the body's tissues of oxygen. Second-hand smoke puts non-smokers at a 25 percent higher risk for developing heart disease, and smoking doubles the risk for stroke. It also blocks pulmonary vessels, causing chronic obstructive pulmonary disease (COPD). Between its negative effects on the heart and the lungs, tobacco use is responsible for roughly 6 million largely preventable deaths per year.

One of the most effective and enjoyable ways to reduce the risk of heart disease (for both prevention and recovery) is walking. While strenuous, quick, competitive, and muscle-building exercise routines often cause damage to body tissues and tax the heart, walking is a paced, effective, and toning way to increase blood circulation, improve digestion through bowel muscle toning, improve respiratory function through increased breathing rate (and fresh air), and strengthen cardiac muscles gradually and with purpose. Most of my clients mention walking along a trail or beach as one of their number one methods for reducing stress. I take my dog walking daily on a nearby system of trails, and the brisk walking makes a big difference in my productivity and state of mind. Try to walk between one and three miles daily, lifting the feet and keeping good posture. Keep the head up and push from the belly and the backs of the thighs. Carry light one-pound weights if desired.

General dietary protocols are easy to follow, inexpensive, and go a long way toward maintaining and supporting a healthy heart. For most adults, the following regimen of foods and supplements will be appropriate for both prevention and recuperation:

- **Remove saturated fats.** Limit consumption of this fat to less than 7 percent of daily calories. Switch saturated fats for yogurt, fruit spreads, or olive oil when cooking or preparing foods.

- **Eliminate hydrogenated oils.** These can cause hardening of the arteries (arteriosclerosis) and the build-up of plaque (athero-sclerosis). Completely avoid these toxic non-food substances at all costs. Look at labels and do not buy any product that lists hydrogenated or partially hydrogenated oil, cottonseed oil, frac-tionated oil, shortening, coconut oil, palm or palm-kernel oils, and monodiglycerides. Consume heart-healthy oils and use flax-seed, evening primrose, borage, and black currant oils. Flaxseed is the best for most people, though evening primrose, borage, and black currant are often advisable for women suffering pre-menstrual syndrome or other hormone disorders, or who are menopausal. Buy flaxseed whole and grind it, storing it in the re-frigerator or freezer. Include it in your meals and as a substitute for butter when baking.

- **Add omega-3 fatty acids.** These reduce the clotting tendency of blood and can reduce the risk of heart attack. Eat salmon and other oily fish, walnuts, and even oregano.

- **Avoid high fructose corn syrup.**

- **Add an abundance of green leafy vegetables to the diet.** These high-fiber and high-folic acid foods support digestion and brain function.

- **Reduce red meat.** The infamous "meat and potatoes" diet is a prime trigger for coronary heart disease, especially if the person smokes or drinks alcohol. Replace it with occasional chicken, turkey, or venison, but let fish be the primary "meat."

- **Cook with garlic and onions.**

- **Adopt and adapt the Mediterranean diet.** At first glance, this region's culinary habits seem high in olive oil, red wine, cheese, bread and tomato sauce, but it's healthy because it features variety and proper portion sizes. French and Italian cuisine center on whole grains, fresh greens, lightly cooked vegetables, and abundant fresh fruit—with pastas, sauces, and desserts featured as special treats and not main courses. Keep the portion sizes of carbohydrates, such as whole grain pasta, to one cup per meal.

- **Drink green tea.** The tea plant *Camellia sinensis* produces all true teas: black, green, white, oolong, etc., and each varies in how it was fermented and processed. Polyphenol-rich green tea is especially useful in a heart-healthy diet (as well as for men with prostate issues) because its catechins (polyphenols) lower cholesterol and enhance the metabolism of lipids, or fats. A natural bitter, green tea can be consumed at one to two cups per day for a lovely drink; I blend mine with spearmint, cardamom and cinnamon for a traditional delicious Moroccan beverage.

- **Include herbs and spices such as** cumin, rosemary, thyme, oregano, sage, lemongrass, lovage and lavender; these add zest and vital phytochemicals to dinners and salsas.

## Cardiotonics and Vascular Tonics

Some herbs have the ability to affect heart tissue operation and rhythm, which likely evolved as protection mechanisms to deter predators. Some of these mechanisms involve making the predator nauseous, or causing the predator to have hallucinations—either way, the predator won't want to snack on that plant again. Some plants cause the predator's heart to race faster—or to stop pumping altogether.

Herbalists have carefully studied these reactions over the centuries and have learned which plants affect the heart. For instance, foxglove (*Digitalis* spp.) is a known cardioactive and curative with very distinct effects—it is not a tonic. Foxglove contains powerful cardiac glycosides that increase the heart's ability to hold on to increased sodium and calcium levels within the cells, enhancing the efficiency and force of the heart's pumping action without increasing its demand for extra oxygen, allowing muscles to be more effective as blood transporters without using undue energy or suffering from a lack of oxygen due to lowered blood pressure or cell membrane permeability. [15] Today, scientists extract or isolate the so-called "pharmaco-active" substance, the cardiac glycoside *digoxin* from the foxglove plant. However, cardiac glycosides have a potential downfall: they are fairly insoluble and are not excreted from the body as quickly as many medical practitioners would like. This can lead to an overly strong pumping action of the heart and possibly death.

Foxglove is an example of a cardioactive plant; it has a direct stimulatory action on the heart or cardiovascular system, and it contains pharmaceutically active cardiac glycosides. This is in contrast to cardiotonics that have no cardiac glycosides and are considered tonic, nourishing, and sustaining to the cardiovascular system and the heart in particular. Safe and common cardiotonics include:

- **hawthorn** (*Crataegus* spp.): Hawthorn is a tree that grows naturally throughout the east coast of the United States, Europe, and elsewhere. Covered with thick spines, the hawthorn tree boasts leaves, flowers, and berries that can all be used medicinally as heart tonics. Hawthorn does not contain cardiac glycosides—instead, its beneficial action on the heart is due to its flavonoids and its oligomeric procyanidins, chemicals that are

---

15   Hoffmann (1996), 2–31.

both antioxidant and anti-inflammatory. The scientific advisory board German Commission E Monograph asserts that hawthorn accomplishes its toning action by increasing coronary and myocardial circulation through a dilation of the coronary arteries. This dilation naturally lowers blood pressure and allows greater circulation throughout the body.

- **linden** (*Tilia europaea*): Containing volatile oils and flavonoids, the flowers of this stately tree (also called lime blossom) are nervine and antispasmodic, which gives it a place in cardio healing. It is also mildly diuretic and anti-inflammatory, making it an ideal long-term cardiotonic for the prevention of heart disease, especially related to stress.

- **motherwort** (*Leonurus cardiaca*): Long revered in Europe and the folk medicine of Russia, motherwort is renowned for two things: (1) aiding congestion of the heart and strengthening heart tone; and (2) acting as a nervine tonic to soothe jangled nerves and even hysteria. Most herbalists today appreciate motherwort for its bitter principle, which lends the herb to use in digestive complaints (especially when prepared as a syrup). Many people find relief using motherwort for congestion in both the pelvic region and the cardiac region, and I've used it countless times for easing nervous tension without sedation. I find motherwort combines well with blue vervain and lemon balm.

- **rose** (*Rosa rugosa*): Rose is listed here as an indirect cardiotonic primarily because of its effects on the nervous system. The hips (those red sacs that appear after the flower falls) are packed with vitamin C that can easily be consumed in a tea, syrup, or jam, and were recommended nearly 2,000 years ago by Dioscorides as a treatment for coughing up blood. For centuries, the petals and unopened buds have been used for syrups and eye washes, and

I find I also use the petals frequently in my herbal formulas for women, for teenagers, and to allay anxiety. Roses, in addition to being the flower of love, are traditionally a calming and palliative remedy for grief and emotional loss, which are the emotions of the heart. Harvest blossoms that have not been sprayed with pesticides or herbicides.

- **oats** (*Avena sativa*): A tonic for the nervous system and herbal remedy for exhaustion, poor fertility, and mineral loss, oatstraw and oats milky tops have long been used traditionally and are now gaining recognition as healthy heart enhancers. Used traditionally to check heart palpitations and improve vessel tone, oats are also valued for their high calcium content (which can strengthen the efficacy of the heart's pumping action) and as a food to reduce cholesterol. A diet high in oats is naturally a fiber-rich diet; use the milky tops as supplementary infusions.

- **ginkgo** (*Ginkgo biloba*): Ginkgo has been studied as a heart-healing herb because it shows remarkable effects in those suffering from heart diseases. Laboratory research has suggested the use of ginkgo in the prevention of coronary thrombosis as well as in the recovery of strokes and heart attacks. It lowers blood pressure and stimulates the flow of blood to the brain and to the periphery of the body, such as hands and feet. Herbalists use ginkgo to restore tone and elasticity to vessel tissues and to improve circulation throughout the body.[16] Combine ginkgo with hawthorn and prickly ash.

Additionally, some herbs are not tonics but are tier 3 corollary herbs to support the cardio system:

---

16   Hoffmann (1996), 2–35.

- **yarrow** (*Achillea millefolium*): a strong vasodilator, yarrow is both diuretic and astringent. It tones the vascular tissues, promotes the free flow of fluids through those vessels, and lowers blood pressure. It is traditionally used to give elasticity and tone to vessel tissues and to improve the flow of blood and other fluids throughout the body, helping to "flush" excess fluid from the body. Yarrow works in different ways based on its preparation: brewing a hot tea of yarrow leaves or flowers will induce sweating (as a diaphoretic), which is helpful during fever. In this capacity, yarrow combines well with elderflower and ginger. Drinking the cold tea stimulates the need to urinate (as a diuretic), which is helpful for urinary tract infection or kidney infection, because the herb is helping to flush out this system (at the same time bringing germ-fighting and astringent properties to the area). Use yarrow in very small doses and combined with other herbs for the heart, such as hawthorn. Its bitterness will naturally suggest a small dose, especially in teas; chewing on fresh leaves is also recommended.

- **prickly ash** (*Zanthoxylum americanum*): the inner bark of this tree restores circulation as a peripheral vasodilator. I often use this herb in cases of cold hands and feet, and it combines well with ginkgo biloba, ginger, and hawthorn.

## High Blood Pressure

Blood pressure is determined by measuring the systolic pressure (when the heart pumps blood through the arteries) and then the diastolic pressure (when the heart rests between beats). Normal blood pressure for infants is generally 90 over 60, written 90/60. Normal blood pressure for adults 120/80, while 140/90 is considered high, though everyone is different and certain conditions, such as diabetes, affect what is considered "normal."

Key risk factors for the development of high blood pressure and hypertension include obesity, the consumption of alcohol over an extended period of time in great quantities, smoking tobacco, genetic predisposition, excessive sodium intake, and stress. Reversing these risk factors is essential in reducing the symptoms of the disease and guarding against the consequences of the disease, which can include stroke, myocardial infarction, embolism, and aneurism, among others. High blood pressure can lead to chronic heart disease, brain damage, kidney (renal) disease and renal failure, and death.

Vasodilator herbs can reduce the stress on the vascular system by increasing the diameter of the vessel and reducing the volume of fluid pumping through the veins, thereby relieving stress on the heart muscle. Some herbs, such as mistletoe, have been used throughout history but lack scientific study; others such as hawthorn are more familiar and demonstrate reliable safety.

Safe tier 1 tonic herbs include all the cardiotonics listed above: hawthorn, motherwort, linden, and ginkgo. Also consider:

- **dandelion** (*Taraxacum officinale*) **leaf:** because dandelion is a diuretic and is high in potassium, it strengthens the vessel walls and reduces pressure on the heart.

- **garlic** (*Allium sativum*) and **mastic** (*Pistacia lentiscus*): reduce cholesterol build-up and blood pressure (see the following entry for cholesterol for more details).

- **prickly ash bark** (*Zanthoxylum* spp.): stimulates circulation.

- **hibiscus** (*Hibiscus rosa-sinensis*) has been shown in a 2008 U.S. Department of Agriculture study to lower blood pressure significantly. [17] In their study, people with mild hypertension who

---

17   Bliss, R. M. (2008).

drank three cups of hibiscus tisane daily were able to lower their blood pressure by 7.2 points compared with a placebo group that lowered only 1.3 points. People with much higher blood pressure realized an even more impressive 13.2 point reduction in their systolic blood pressure and a diastolic reduction of 6.4 points. Hibiscus makes a tart and tangy addition to many teas and can be considered a healthy addition especially for those wanting to add its gentle benefits to their cardiac care strategy.

- **rue** (*Ruta graveolens*): Rue is a common garden herb renowned for its bitter principles. It contains heart-friendly flavonoids including quercetin and rutin, as well as coumarins. It's a powerful emmenagogue and abortifacient, so keep this in mind when working with women who may be or may wish to soon become pregnant. Rue is traditionally used in very small doses to increase peripheral circulation and lower elevated blood pressure.

## *High Blood Pressure Formulas*
### A FORMULA FOR HIGH BLOOD PRESSURE

> › 2 parts hawthorn

> › 2 parts linden

> › 2 parts dandelion leaf

> › 1 part oatstraw or oats milky tops

### ANOTHER FORMULA FOR HIGH BLOOD PRESSURE

> › 2 parts hibiscus

> › 1 part hawthorn

> › 1 part linden

> › 1 part motherwort

## Low Blood Pressure (Hypotension) and Poor Circulation

Medically, low blood pressure is diagnosed by a systolic/diastolic reading of 90/60 with no symptoms. Hypotension presents with inadequate blood flow, poor circulation, light-headedness, dizziness, nausea, and/or foggy thinking. It often reveals itself when a person stands up from a seated or supine position and suddenly feels faint. Low blood pressure is not considered a problem if it is a life-long reading of blood pressure at low numbers, but it is advisable to monitor the condition to guard against acute hypotension.

Risk factors and causes include pregnancy, certain medications and drugs, severe injury and loss of blood, dehydration, allergic reaction to medication, food, or alcohol (anaphylactic shock), heart arrhythmias, heat exhaustion, and liver disease.

A number of drugs can induce a state of hypotension, especially drugs that (directly or indirectly) affect the contractility of the heart and lower blood pressure or rhythm; these drugs can include high blood pressure medications, diuretics, antipsychotics, anti-anxiety drugs, and antidepressants. Similarly, taking a diuretic herb such as dandelion can exacerbate hypotension.

There are few herbal vasoconstrictors, though astringents are often helpful:

- **Scotch broom** (*Sarothamnus scoparius*) and **butcher's-broom** (*Ruscus aculeatus*): Hoffmann lists both brooms as vasoconstrictors.[18] Scotch broom is an invasive flowering legume and butcher's-broom is an evergreen shrub nicknamed "knee holly." Butcher's-broom may contain heart-affecting glycosides; Hoffmann lists Scotch broom as the safest example of a vasoconstrictor that raises blood pressure slightly due to its vasoconstricting action but notes that its most common application is topically on hemorrhoids.

---

18   Hoffmann (1996).

- **yarrow** (*Achillea millefolium*): diuretic and diaphoretic; yarrow can be an occasional tier 3 corollary herb for low blood pressure and vessel tone.

- **cranesbill** (*Geranium maculatum*): a gentle astringent, cranesbill is applied topically to swollen vessels and hemorrhoids; can be taken as a tea for chronic hypotension.

- **horse chestnut** (*Aesculus hippocastanum*) appears to strengthen and tone vessel tissues themselves, possibly because of its saponins and glycosides. It is best used in cases of "congestion" of the cardiovascular system that is impeding proper blood flow and leading to hypotension. Butcher's-broom is used in a similar manner.

Warming herbs and spices may help improve circulation. These include:

- **black tea** (*Camellia sinensis*): In a U.S. Department of Agriculture study, researchers found black tea drinkers lowered their blood lipid levels by 6 to 10 percent in a relatively short length of time (three weeks) using five servings of tea per day. [19]

- **wild sarsaparilla** (*Aralia nudicaulis*): the root provides a "yang" energizing effect yet is much milder than black tea and contains no caffeine.

- **peppermint** (*Mentha × piperita*):promotes circulation to the periphery and may have a mild constricting action on the blood vessels; stronger than spearmint, which tends to direct its action to the digestive system and the brain, peppermint tends to direct its action outward, relieving cold hands and feet.

---

19   Bliss, R. M. (2003).

- **cayenne** (*Capsicum annuum*): warming spices such as hot pepper, ginger, cinnamon, and cardamom can stimulate blood flow, though they are not necessarily vasoconstrictors or astringents; their warming action can be used as an "energizing" effect for hypotension sufferers with depleted energy, nausea, or light-headedness.

### Low Blood Pressure (Hypotension) and Poor Circulation Formulas
#### A FORMULA FOR LOW BLOOD PRESSURE

> › 2 parts oatstraw or oats milky tops
>
> › 1 part cranesbill
>
> › 1 part motherwort
>
> › ½ part peppermint

#### A FORMULA FOR POOR CIRCULATION TO THE PERIPHERY

> › 2 parts garlic
>
> › 1 part prickly ash
>
> › 1 part wild sarsaparilla
>
> › 1 part peppermint or cayenne

## Cholesterol and Atherosclerosis

The condition of having high cholesterol levels in the arteries and vessels is known as hypercholesterolemia, a serious issue that can cause heart disease and stroke. Cholesterol is a perfectly normal substance—rather waxy and fatty, named from the Greek *chole-* (bile) and *stereos* (solid)—and it's produced in our livers and found in the foods we eat. We need some cholesterol to synthesize vitamin D and to achieve proper function of our bodily systems; steroid hormones, such as testosterone and cortisol that are manufactured in the adrenal cortex and the gonads, for example, can only be manufactured from cholesterol.

But too much cholesterol is not good; it builds up in our blood vessels and arteries, and since it's waxy and doesn't wash away with the flow of blood, but instead sticks to vessel walls, it builds up over time. The thickening of arteries due to this plaque build-up is called atherosclerosis—this is different from arteriolosclerosis, which is the hardening of the vessel walls themselves. Plaque build-up leads to a smaller opening through which blood can flow, forcing the heart to pump harder and leading to high blood pressure. Caucasians typically suffer more cholesterol symptoms (and therefore more gallbladder and gallstone issues) since the antioxidant melatonin is believed to enhance the conversion of cholesterol to bile. As a result, fewer people of color experience gallstones and other cholesterol-related illness.

Plants contain cholesterol-like substances called phytosterols, which are virtually identical to human cholesterol. Since the cholesterol we produce in our livers is shunted into the digestive system and then recycled and sent back to the livers to be used again, the presence of plant-derived phytosterols tricks the body into utilizing phytosterols instead, excreting the excess through the feces. This reduces the amount of cholesterol the body believes it needs to make, which results in lower cholesterol in our bloodstreams. Taking advantage of these phytosterols is a common-sense approach to reducing cholesterol levels in the body. Plants with ideal phytosterol chemistry include vegetable oils and nuts.

Supplements for the reduction of symptoms of atherosclerosis include niacin (though this one is controversial and, for the herbalist, not a holistic method), as well as omega-3 fatty acids and vitamin C. To obtain these last two, consume salt-water fish with meals and vitamin C–rich foods and herbs, such as lemon, lime, watercress, spinach, rose hips, and sorrel.

Herbs that support the reduction of cholesterol include:

- **oats** (*Avena sativa*): Research has shown that consumption of oats reduces the inflammation associated with atherosclerosis. [20]

- **mastic** (*Pistacia lentiscus*): known for its ability to kill *Helicobacter pylori* and thereby relieve symptoms of peptic ulcer, mastic also reduces cholesterol. The sticky mastic resin has long been chewed to ease stomachache and it has received much attention for its ability to absorb cholesterol and thereby lower blood pressure and reduce the risk of consequent heart failure. [21]

- **garlic** (*Allium sativum*): widely regarded as the first protocol for naturally remedying hypercholesterolemia and atherosclerosis, garlic reduces hyperlipidemia, hypertension, and thrombus formation, guarding against thrombosis or blood clots in the blood vessels. Garlic has even been shown to be preventative, being successfully employed before atherosclerotic symptoms appear. It can reduce lipid content in the cells of arteries and even prevent this lipid, or fatty cell, accumulation.

## *Cholesterol and Atherosclerosis Formulas*
### A Formula for High Cholesterol or Atherosclerosis

> › 2 parts hawthorn

> › 2 parts oatstraw or oats milky tops

> › 1 part garlic

> › 1 part rose hips

### Another Formula for High Cholesterol or Atherosclerosis

> › 2 parts hawthorn

> › 1 part mastic

---

20   Behall and Hallfrisch (2006).

21   Kartalis, Didagelos, and Georgiadis (2016).

> › 1 part garlic

> › 1 part ginkgo

## Pre- and Post-Stroke and Heart Attack Strategies

If ever there was an opportunity to reverse disease and illness based on simple lifestyle changes, heart health is it. The heart and entire cardio-vascular system responds readily to changes in the diet—both positively and negatively, and our choices make a world of difference in current and future heart health. Eating less, stopping smoking, eating less fatty and fried foods, and walking daily have an enormous positive impact on the structure and function of the heart and vascular system. Without these positive lifestyle choices, diseases can result:

- **Stroke** refers to a blocked blood vessel or bleeding in the brain that results in brain damage. Medical personnel distinguish be-tween severe strokes and "mini" strokes, each indicating that the circulatory system has just malfunctioned and the brain is in dan-ger. Symptoms include weakness, numbness, blurry vision, confu-sion, difficulty speaking, inability to process information, speaking of people not present as if they were present, etc. These indicate an immediate emergency; proceed to the emergency room.

- **Heart attack**, also called myocardial infarction, happens when blood flow to the heart has suspended long enough to cause damage to the heart tissue and temporarily or permanently in-terrupt its pumping rhythm. Most heart attacks are caused by blood clots that block one of the coronary arteries, and these blood clots, in turn, can be caused by a build-up of plaque or cholesterol on the artery's walls.

- **Thrombosis** is the obstruction of a vessel or artery (vascular oc-clusion) at the point where a blood clot forms.

- **Embolism** is the obstruction of a vessel or artery by a blockage (vascular occlusion) of clotted blood that has broken free from its point of origin and has traveled to a distant part of the body, potentially lodging in a random vessel or artery and depriving that section of the body (and eventually) the heart and brain of oxygen.

- **Aneurism** is the swelling and ballooning of a blood vessel that can rupture.

- **Angina pectoris** is a warning sign that one of these cardiovascular illnesses is about to occur. Angina pectoris occurs when a compromised or sick heart is pushed past capacity due to over-exertion (such as shoveling snow off the sidewalk or running to catch a missed flight). The over-stressed heart muscle has to work much harder and faster but without the necessary oxygen. The pain causes people to believe they are having a heart attack.

Obviously, stroke, heart attack, embolism, and aneurism are dire medical emergencies and I make no claims here to treat any of these conditions. What we can do, however, is provide herbs and dietary and lifestyle guidance to help prevent these occurrences from happening in the first place, as well as herbal support to strengthen the cardiovascular system in particular in a preventive and supportive fashion. Healing arts professionals can help their clients at risk for stroke, heart attack, embolism, or aneurism (either because of genetic predisposition, smoking, alcoholism, poor mobility, high cholesterol, or previous history with weakened arteries or vessels) by encouraging them to follow the following formulary program as a beginning point for reducing that risk. Educate your clients about reversing poor lifestyle choices in favor of heart-healthy choices. Your goal should be to support the body in its efforts to strengthen capillary and vessel walls, to reduce plaque build-up and lower cholesterol, to improve flow of blood through the system through physical exercise and mobility, and to strengthen the heart's pumping action and its efficacy in transporting oxygenated blood through the core and to the periphery. Follow the dietary and supplement guidance in the Cholesterol section (using food and diet as medicine), slowly adding herbal remedies such as teas, tinctures, or capsules over time.

### *Pre- and Post-Stroke and Heart Attack Formulas*
#### A FORMULA FOR PREVENTIVE HEART CARE

> › 2 parts linden flower
>
> › 1 part oatstraw or oats milky tops
>
> › 1 part spearmint
>
> › 1 part rose hips

#### A FORMULA FOR PREVENTIVE HEART CARE

> › 2 parts hawthorn
>
> › 1 part linden
>
> › 1 part garlic
>
> › 1 part oatstraw or oats milky tops

#### A FORMULA TO STRENGTHEN BLOOD VESSELS

> › 2 parts hawthorn
>
> › 1 part motherwort
>
> › 1 part prickly ash
>
> › 1 part nettle

#### A FORMULA FOR POST-HEART ATTACK CARE

> › 2 parts hawthorn
>
> › 2 parts oatstraw or oats milky tops

- › 1 part khella
- › 1 part night blooming cereus (cactus, *Selenicereus grandiflorus*)
- › 1 part garlic or ginger

### A FORMULA FOR POST ANGINA PECTORIS

- › 2 parts ginkgo
- › 2 parts hawthorn
- › 1 part yarrow
- › 1 part motherwort

### ANOTHER FORMULA FOR POST ANGINA PECTORIS

- › 2 parts oats or oats milky tops
- › 2 parts hawthorn
- › 1 part prickly ash
- › 1 part garlic

## Grief and Heartache

Heartache is an emotional condition but throughout Western history it has been associated with the organ in our chests that pumps blood. Rightly or wrongly, this connection has bequeathed herbal heritage with many plant-based remedies, liqueurs, and beverages that help the heart and bear names linking the cardiac muscle with love, affection, and friendship. For instance, the herb motherwort is *Leonurus cardiaca*, or "heart of the lion," alluding to its traditional use in formulas that give a person courage as well as in formulas that literally strengthen the heart. (It may also allude to a mother's large heart, as this is an herb given to mothers of young children who demonstrate unconditional love). The medieval drink, the cordial, was also named for its cardiovascular strengthening properties, and Welsh herbalist David Hoffmann notes that borage was the herb of choice in first preparing cordials (etymologically related to *courage*) because this herb was known to give people "heart." [22] A quick look in the dictionary shows that the word *cordial* is now associated with sincerity and deep emotion, warmth and geniality, though its original sense of "relating to the heart" is diminishing.

Heartache and sadness of the heart have been poetically recounted for centuries in ballads, love-songs and sonnets, and healers have long offered solace to the bereaved. Having heart, falling in love, bearing something courageously, and feeling your heart burst from anguish or sadness are all expressions we use to connect our emotions with the heart. Whether or not science will one day confirm that the heart has something to do with our deepest inner emotions remains to be seen. But our herbal tradition offers a great deal of warmth and medicine to alleviate all conditions of the heart: physical, emotional, or spiritual.

Grief is one of those conditions, and it has profound physiological consequences on the body. The sadness of losing someone or something of great meaning in one's life can be devastating, leading to depression, suicidal feelings, remorse, guilt, a "heavy heart," and the separation of oneself from a community of people who could help. Loss can be excruciating, and of course there is no magic herb that will return those we have lost. A centeredness in spirituality and a familiarity with cycles can begin to bring about a sense of understanding and acceptance of death, knowing (with both mind and heart) that death is part of life. It's such an emotional concept that it hardly makes cognitive sense when we're experiencing a good day, so it's generally very difficult to grasp when we're bereaved, but it's worth noting that a spiritual approach to grief, loss, death, and transition (as opposed to a pharmaceutical approach) is the most genuine and enduring way to find peace.

---

22   Hoffmann (1996), 2–31.

In this context, there are a few special herbs that have long been part of this process, and how you use them is up to you. British herbalist Anne McIntyre once said it doesn't matter how you use them—whether as teas, tinctures, powders, etc.—as long as you connect with them. A spiritual connection is encouraged here, which is a longstanding traditional tenet of herbal medicine alongside its pharmacological aspects.

- **rose** (*Rosa rugosa, R.* spp.): the scent of roses and their feel, taste, and energy all combine to provide a lasting and visceral feeling of release from states of debilitating grief. The rose has a special place in herbal therapy for grief, sadness, depression, and especially bereavement; they are also versatile and can be used in a myriad of ways, including being steeped in massage oil, taken as a syrup, drunk as a tea, chewed fresh, infused in a bath, infused in honey, and inhaled as an essential oil.

- **motherwort** (*Leonurus cardiaca*): long used to help mothers deal with the complex and chaotic mayhem resulting from the stress of raising young children. Encourage clients to chew the leaves for a bitter yet strengthening burst of energy, or take the tincture at signs of feeling overwhelmed, stressed, sad, or when they're grieving the loss of a part of themselves—such as their freedom or youth.

- **lemon** (*Citrus × limon*), lemon verbena (*Aloysia citrodora*), and lemon balm (*Melissa officinalis*): use these to awaken and refresh after a period of mourning. Bright, citrusy, lemony flavors wake up the spirit and open the eyes. Drinking lemon teas can warm the heart, revive the spirit, and boost energy.

Other traditional herbs for grief include borage, violet, mullein, St. John's wort, basil, spearmint, holy basil (tulsi), lemongrass, and the heart herb hawthorn.

*Grief and Heartache Formulas*
### A FORMULA FOR GRIEF (AS A TEA OR HONEY)

> › 2 parts rose

> › 1 part hawthorn

> › 1 part lemon balm

> › 1 part St. John's wort

### ANOTHER FORMULA FOR GRIEF (AS A TINCTURE)

> › 2 parts motherwort

> › 1 part skullcap

> › 1 part wild sarsaparilla

> › 1 part rose

### A FORMULA FOR OPENING UP TO LOVE (AS A TEA OR HOT COCOA)

> › 2 parts rose

> › 1 part ashwagandha

> › 1 part cocoa

> › 1 part rhodiola

# Headache and Migraine

We'll end this chapter on the care of the cardiovascular system with a discussion of headaches. There are two primary types of headaches: tension and vascular (or migraine). Tension headaches are often caused by stress or emotional irritation, which lead to involuntary muscular constriction in the neck and shoulder and results in aches in the head, neck, shoulders, and eye pain. Migraines, however, appear to be related to involuntary blood vessel constriction in the brain and are notoriously difficult to treat with herbs, as few herbs are strong enough to eradicate migraines, and those that are can be dangerous to use, especially for those suffering from chronic and frequent migraines. Therefore the recommendations here are primarily for mild-to-moderate tension headaches. Headaches can be triggered by an allergic reaction to food, spinal damage that needs correction, hormonal imbalance, illness (influenza or other viral infection), constipation, liver obstruction, Lyme infection, addictive substance withdrawal, dehydration, and as the result of cleanses or certain weight-loss diets.

Encourage clients to discover the cause of their headaches. Often this is easy (maybe they fought with someone or participated in an irritating meeting), but sometimes it's not obvious. Did they eat a disagreeable food? Explore their diet and check for other symptoms present in the body. Have they been bitten by a tick? In New England among other locales, headaches and muscle aches are red flags to look for the typical red bull's-eye of an infected tick bite. What about their normal routine? Is there a new diet or medication? Finally, don't ignore headaches reported by children; though they may be pleas for attention, chronic headaches in children could indicate an emergency condition and should be addressed. For an occasional tension headache, suggest the following:

- **Go to sleep.** The body can heal itself if given the time.

- **Take a warm bath** with lavender, passionflower, lemon balm, rose petals, or chamomile in the bathwater, tied in a muslin bag and held under the faucet.

- **Rub the shoulders and loosen the neck muscles** with simple head roll exercises. Stretch the arms out to the side, swing the body to loosen muscles, and go for a walk in the fresh air.

- **Gently rub** lavender, rose, or chamomile-infused oil onto the temples and wrists.

- **Drink plenty of fresh water** and **turn off** the lights

When a headache is caused by the constriction of blood vessels, part of the therapy can involve "opening" up those vessels so proper blood flow can resume. The formula should include nervine tonics, analgesics, circulatory tonics, and any other corollary support herbs needed. Analgesics lessen or even eliminate pain, especially if corollary actions are taken to mitigate the causes. Choose tier 1 tonics (primarily nervines), tier 2 Specifics (primarily analgesics), and then tier 3 corollary herbs, perhaps antispasmodics for muscle tension or bitters for digestion. Cardiovascular tonics such as ginger can both relieve stagnant congestion and stimulate digestion. The best tier 4 vehicle is traditionally feverfew, which has a folk use of numbing headaches and encouraging blood flow to the brain. Other tier 4 vehicles that increase blood flow to the brain include ginkgo (*Ginkgo biloba*) and gotu kola (*Centella asiatica*).

### Headache and Migraine Formulas

#### A FORMULA FOR A MILD TENSION HEADACHE

> › 2 parts skullcap
>
> › 1 part willow
>
> › 1 part lavender
>
> › 1 part feverfew

#### ANOTHER FORMULA FOR A MILD TENSION HEADACHE

> › 2 parts holy basil (tulsi)
>
> › 1 part meadowsweet
>
> › 1 part Jamaican dogwood
>
> › 1 part ginkgo

## A Formula for a Vascular Headache

> › 2 parts sage
>
> › 1 part lavender
>
> › 1 part turmeric
>
> › 1 part oats milky tops

The cardiovascular system is one of the most intricate, the most read-ily influenced, and one of the most treatable systems of the body. Despite its importance, I encourage you to feel confident in working within the parameters of this book to positively support the structure and function of the heart muscle and vascular system. Our heritage of herbal healing for the heart is vast, well-documented, and accessible, with many of the most profound cardiotonics being easy to obtain or grow. Care for the heart is a sacred responsibility as well as a practical goal; using the tonic herbs in this chapter as well as dietary and lifestyle changes or management are the best ways to advance the health of these organs and live long into the future.

# CHAPTER FIVE

# Respiratory

Herbal medicine has long had a strong tradition of caring for the respiratory system—both the upper respiratory tract (the sinuses and throat) and the lower respiratory (the lungs). Because some herbs have very distinct and noticeable effects (such as drying up mucus secretions, causing bronchial muscle contractions, easing contractions, and soothing wet or dry coughs), their use has long been documented historically, and there is much information and experience throughout many cultures for treating respiratory ailments with plants.

Many of the respiratory remedies are fragile plants found in fragile habitats; please refer to Glossary E at the back of this book for the at-risk and to-watch lists prepared by United Plant Savers, an organization dedicated to the preservation of medicinal plants. On these lists are many of the herbs we consider primary upper and lower respiratory herbs, including pleurisy root, osha, echinacea, goldenseal, lomatium, eyebright, and wild indigo. If you must use them, do so respectfully, minimally, and carefully.

# Upper Respiratory Tract

The upper respiratory system comprises primarily the ears, nose, and throat. Due to their tiny structures, narrow passageways, proximity to each other, and strong influence from environmental triggers, such as allergens and toxins, the ears, nose, and throat can be quick to succumb to congestion and infection. Ear infections in babies and toddlers are common due to the incomplete formation of the structures and the easily inflamed tissues. Sinus congestion and infection, such as sinusitis, obstruct breathing and diminish oxygen supply and also contribute to secondary infections and issues such as sore throat, irritated sinus tissues (internally and externally), cough, headache, blurry vision, and even nausea. Ear, nose, and throat infections can be caused variously by viruses, bacteria, and fungi. A clinical diagnosis is essential before moving forward in herbal treatment, since certain conditions (such as strep throat) can become severe and cause serious bodily damage if not treated with allopathic measures such as antibiotics.

Since there are many different viral, bacterial, and fungal infections that can cause aggravation in the ear, nose, and throat, we'll address these issues by action needed, since one action may address a variety of causes. Keep in mind that the upper respiratory system is, like all other systems, connected to the rest of the body and will therefore have long-reaching effects; for instance, sinus congestion can lead to lower respiratory illness and even cardiac illness, just as ear infections can affect balance and central nervous system function. Always address with the actions needed but remember to address the whole person and not just the symptom, using tonic herbs to strengthen as your tier 1 foundation.

## Ear

While the outer structure, or auricle of the ear, seems relatively simple in its design for collecting and amplifying sound, the inner structure is quite complex. In simple terms, sound waves are corralled through the external auditory canal, past the ear drum (the tympanic membrane), and through a fluid-filled cavity studded with sensitive hairs that send nerve impulses to a portion of the cerebral cortex. Here, sound waves are deciphered and sound is "heard," with some sort of meaning attached to the sound wave.

The three tiny bones of the middle ear (the malleus, incus, and stapes) are perfectly situated so that movement of the ear drum causes a chain reaction that ends with the movement of fluid in the cochlea of the inner ear. This fluid can become inflamed due to physical pressure or through bacterial or viral infection.

The goals of the herbalist begin with addressing the person as a whole person, not just an ear or a symptom. Ask: Is stress a contributing factor? Are the lower respiratory or cardiac systems in need? Is blood flow carrying oxygen to the brain normally?

Comfort from pain is important, so analgesics should be considered for both external and internal relief. Finally, diet should be considered, as certain foods may "clog" the system while others will open it up. Dairy is often a culprit in high-mucus conditions and congestion, while warming carminative foods such as cayenne, cardamom, clove, ginger, horseradish, hot peppers, and other spices can speed blood flow and open vessels that were otherwise clogged.

Obviously, ear obstruction due to physical causes such as wax buildup or an object embedded in the ear require assistance other than that which herbs can provide. See a doctor when necessary. Some of the actions needed in treatment of ear problems:

### Antibacterial
Specific antibacterial herbs can fight the infection both internally and externally:

- **garlic** (*Allium sativum*): fresh garlic, taken internally, is a mainstay for fighting both upper and lower respiratory infections. Garlic contains allicin, a potent antioxidant. Never insert garlic cloves in the ear canal.

- **goldenseal** (*Hydrastis canadensis*): the root is a powerful antibacterial and antifungal usually taken as a powder or tincture. It is also bitter (stimulating the digestive system) and is very astringent (drying up catarrh or mucus in both the upper and lower respiratory systems). Do not use goldenseal if you are pregnant or nursing (it is contraindicated in breastfeeding because its astringent action will dry up the breast milk). Goldenseal capsules can be taken internally to fight ear infection or drops of tincture or oil can be applied to a cotton ball and inserted into the outer ear canal.

- **echinacea** (*Echinacea purpurea, E. angustifolia*): especially valuable when the cause of ear infection is viral. Echinacea can be taken as a tea, capsule or tincture internally and also applied to a cotton ball and carefully inserted into the outer ear canal.

### Demulcents and Anti-Inflammatories

Calming, soothing herbs can alleviate pressure, burning, and pain in the ear canal when rubbed on the skin outside the ear and around the neck.

- **mullein** (*Verbascum thapsus*): A primary herb for soothing the lungs, both the leaves and flowers are used. Mullein leaf tea can be drunk for its nervine action, and mullein flowers are infused in olive oil with the warm extract being dropped into the ear canal. Mullein leaf is a specific for calming coughs and spasms of the lower respiratory tract, so it is a good overlap herb when there are infections in both systems.

- **St. John's wort** (*Hypericum perforatum*): antiviral and antibacterial, *Hypericum* is normally used in cases of ear infection to soothe inflamed tissues. St. John's wort can be taken as a tea or capsule internally or infused into an oil to drop into the ear canal or to massage around the ear and neck.

### Warming Herbs

Warming herbs can be made into liniments that are carefully massaged onto the skin around the ear and neck, being sure to avoid sensitive tissues and the eyes. Rubbing these herbs can help stimulate blood flow to the area and can act as a sort of "urtication" with a rubefacient effect, which can be helpful for stagnant conditions such as arthritis. Be sure to watch for inflammation and don't use these herbs in cases of fever or heat; rather, they are beneficial in cold, clammy, and congested cases where the ear canal is "clogged." Consider wintergreen, cinnamon, birch, and peppermint.

### Vehicle

Carrier herbs that have an "affinity" for a particular organ or region of the body can help direct or "usher" the medicinal herbs toward that region. The effect of these tier 4 vehicle herbs will be most appreciated in internal formulas:

- **cleavers** (*Galium aparine*): an herb specific to the lymph system and to increase "flow" all over the body. I've found them particularly useful for the throat, head, and urinary system, and I include cleavers in immune support formulas.

- **horseradish** (*Armoracia rusticana*): Very warming and too stimulating for many children, horseradish quickly opens nasal passage and can be used in small doses as a vehicle in formulas for ear infections. Use common sense with this herb and start minimally.

- **gotu kola** (*Centella asiatica*): traditionally used to promote blood flow to the brain. This nervine herb is a good choice in cases where chronic stress is a factor in ear infection.

- **ginkgo** (*Ginkgo biloba*): ginkgo has been clinically shown to increase blood flow all over the body, including the periphery.

### *Ear Formulas*

#### A FORMULA FOR EAR INFECTION
#### (AS AN INFUSED OIL DROPPED INTO THE EAR CANAL)

> › 2 parts mullein leaf

> › 1 part echinacea

> › 1 part ginkgo

> › 1 part cleavers

#### A FORMULA FOR EAR INFECTION (AS AN INFUSED OIL RUBBED ONTO THE NECK)

> › 1 part St. John's wort

> › 1 part peppermint

#### A FORMULA FOR EAR INFECTION
#### (AS AN INFUSED OIL DROPPED INTO THE EAR CANAL)

> › 2 parts garlic

> › 2 parts mullein flower

> › 1 part echinacea

## Nose

Congestion is the build-up of catarrh, or mucous secretions, that normally help expel toxins or foreign matter from the nasal passages. During infection, there is an over-production of catarrh, a decrease in the efficacy of expulsion, dehydration, and inflammation. Sinusitis refers to viral, fungal, or bacterial infection in the sinus cavity. The following actions will address issues and infections resulting from bacterial, fungal or viral microbes as well as allergic reactions and hay fever.

## Astringent and Anti-Catarrhal

Many astringent herbs are tier 2 Specifics for the upper and lower respiratory systems. Astringent herbs already mentioned include sage, cranesbill, goldenseal, yarrow, and shepherd's purse. Also consider:

- **eyebright** (*Euphrasia* spp.): traditionally used to dry up sinus congestion and clear eyes damaged by smoke; used as a tea internally and a rinse externally.

## Demulcent

Just as emollient herbs soothe inflamed or dry tissue topically, demulcent herbs soothe internally and are generally cooling and mucilaginous for inflamed respiratory or digestive organs.

- **plantain** (*Plantago major, P. lanceolata*): the leaves are demulcent and make an excellent tea taken internally for soothing hot, inflamed, crusty, dry, sore, and aggravated sinus tissues. Combine with mullein leaf and mallow root for a tea or capsule.

## Antispasmodic

Spasmolytic or antispasmodic herbs are helpful for itchy noses and acute sneezing.

- **hyssop** (*Hyssopus officinalis*): widely used in cases of cold and flu as an expectorant and antispasmodic. It is a tier 2 specific for cases of chronic catarrh and long-term upper respiratory infection. Best taken as a hot tea.

- **elecampane** (*Inula helenium*): though it is usually used more for coughs than sinus congestion, it can reduce spasms in the lungs and provide for restful sleep in cases of post-nasal drip.

## Anti-Inflammatory

Reducing inflammation of the sinus cavity is key.

- **St. John's wort** (*Hypericum perforatum*): traditionally used as an anti-inflammatory for the sinuses, this nervine tonic can also be applied topically to sore noses.

- **willow** (*Salix* spp.) and **meadowsweet** (*Filipendula ulmaria*): these salicylate-containing anti-inflammatories can relieve pressure and ease pain both topically and internally.

## Antibacterial, Antifungal

- **garlic** (*Allium sativum*): the sulfur-containing bulb is strongly antimicrobial and also diaphoretic, making it useful for cases of sinusitis with fever. It fights viral and bacterial infection and is effective against intestinal parasites. Because the volatile oil is excreted through the lungs (we can readily smell garlic on the breath) it is a natural bronchial and respiratory tier 2 specific, especially in cases of congestion, catarrh, and cough. (Never insert a garlic clove into the nose.)

- **goldenseal** (*Hydrastis canadensis*): very astringent, goldenseal root powder dries up mucous secretions, teary eyes, sniffles, and weepy congestion. Contraindicated in breastfeeding.

- **osha** (*Ligusticum porteri*): this powerful mucilage-rich, decongestant root with immune-stimulating qualities is extremely difficult to cultivate, which is why it's listed on the United Plant Savers At-Risk List (see glossary E).

- **thyme** (*Thymus vulgaris*): this strong antimicrobial herb is useful for both upper and lower respiratory infections. Use it as a short-term tier 2 specific in tincture form.

## Antiviral

Many herbs offer antibacterial activity, but a few are noted antivirals and can be effective for sinus infection due to colds or other viruses, notably influenza. In addition to St. John's wort, lemon balm, echinacea, and astragalus, consider:

- **elderberry** (*Sambucus nigra*): *in vitro* studies show standardized elderberry liquid extract "exerts in vitro antiviral effects against" both the influenza A and B viruses and other respiratory bacterial pathogens. [23] Herbal heritage uses both elderberry and elderflower to support the immune system, with elderberry being used more for lower respiratory complaints and elderflower used for upper (sinus) issues.

## Warming and Stimulant

For catarrhal conditions, yarrow is a choice herb, as it is astringent, warming, and bitter. Yarrow is frequently included in cold and flu formulas for tinctures, capsules, powders, and teas, though the infusion is bitter. Other warming stimulants include horseradish root, mustard, peppermint, sage, ginger, cayenne, and eucalyptus.

## Alterative

Those herbs that help the body expel wastes from the body (especially via the liver, bladder and kidneys) are alterative. The best for upper respiratory infection include the already mentioned echinacea, garlic, and goldenseal, as well as:

- **cleavers** (*Galium aparine*): because they assist with lymphatic drainage, cleavers are traditionally used in any instance where waste is being excreted (especially for hormonal issues, drug and pharmaceutical use, eczema, and psoriasis, etc.).

---

23   Krawitz, Mraheil, and Stein (2011).

- **red clover** (*Trifolium pratense*): used in folklore as an alterative, red clover is known as a cardioprotective and chemoprotective herb and for its protective effects against cancer. Red clover also reduces cholesterol in men and is used to support women during menopause. [24]

### *Nose Formulas*

#### A FORMULA FOR SINUS CONGESTION (AS A TEA, TINCTURE, OR CAPSULE)

> 2 parts elderflower

> 1 part elderberry

> 1 part yarrow

> 1 part sage

> ½ to 1 part horseradish

#### A FORMULA FOR SINUS CONGESTION WITH INFECTION (AS A TINCTURE)

> 2 parts yarrow

> 1 part sage

> 1 part garlic

> 1 part cleavers (add to ½ cup citrus juice with ¼ teaspoon cayenne powder)

## Throat

Nourishing a sore throat requires all of the herbs listed for the nose as well as some demulcent herbs that can be sucked as lozenges. These include:

---

24    Thompson Healthcare Inc. (2007), 695.

## Demulcent

- **slippery elm** (*Ulmus fulva* or *U. rubra*): This soothing, lubricating and nourishing inner bark can be powdered and eaten, sipped in a tea, or sucked on as a lozenge.

- **comfrey leaf** (*Symphytum officinale*): usually used externally, comfrey is also valuable for regenerating bone tissue growth and as a demulcent for irritating coughs.

- **licorice** (*Glycyrrhiza glabra*): a primary decongestant and demulcent for the lower respiratory system, licorice is smooth and soothing on the throat and can be sipped warm throughout the day. Contraindicated in heart disease and hypertension.

## Throat Formulas

### A Formula for Sore Throat (as a tea or lozenge)

› 2 parts licorice

› 1 part mullein

› 1 part slippery elm

› 1 part plantain

# Lower Respiratory Tract

The lower respiratory tract refers to the trachea, the two bronchial tubes (connecting the esophagus to each lung), and the lungs, which rest inside the pleural cavity. The primary issues affecting the lower respiratory tract include inflammation, infection, and cancer.

- **lung cancer:** The most fatal type of cancer, lung cancer can either originate in the lungs or metastasize there, and is almost always caused by first-hand or second-hand cigarette smoke.[25] It is widely prevalent in coal miners and those exposed to radiation. If a pleural biopsy indicates carcinoma, the person may consider a range of treatments, including surgery, radiation, and chemotherapy. Herbal therapy can be a successful adjunct treatment for symptoms associated with the cancer (which can include coughing blood, shortness of breath, facial nerve issues, throat soreness, joint pain, and general debility).

- **pneumonia:** The most common form of lower respiratory infection, bacterial pneumonia is the most serious, though pneumonia can also be caused by fungi microbes and viruses. Viral bacteria is the most common form in children. The biggest culprit is the germ *Streptococcus pneumoniae*, which causes the lungs to fill with fluid and mucus so the cilia cannot move and lung function is compromised. The illness requires expectorant, alterative, anti-inflammatory, and antimicrobial herbs, among others.

- **tuberculosis:** Caused by an airborne bacteria. The sanitoriums of the Appalachian Mountains were popular in the early twentieth century as a place where people suffering with tuberculosis, or "consumption," could "take the air" and improve their lung function.

- **COPD:** Chronic obstructive pulmonary disease includes, among other diseases, chronic asthmic bronchitis and emphysema. These block airflow on the exhalation making breathing difficult.

---

25   Smoking and Tobacco Use (2004).

- **asthma:** Many triggers can cause acute and chronic asthma, which constricts the chest muscles and reduces airflow to the bronchioles, or can make the bronchial tubes constrict. Triggers include dust mites, animal dander, pollen, and tobacco smoke. (See khella on page 115.)

- **bronchitis:** Inflammation of the two large bronchial tubes that connect the lungs to the windpipe.

- **emphysema:** This is a lower respiratory infection caused by environmental toxins and inhaled toxins such as tobacco smoke. Destroys alveoli and lung tissue: cause shortness of breath and sometimes hyperventilation. Stress on entire body. Less oxygen is introduced to the body and a build-up of carbon monoxide can occur.

- **pleurisy:** In folk medicine, pleurisy referred to any infection of the lungs, but today it refers to inflammation of the pleura, the lining of the pleural cavity that surrounds the lungs.

- **respiratory syncytial virus (RSV):** Common in infants and young children, this viral infection can best be treated with herbs through the mother's breast milk if the child is still breastfeeding, or with glycerite tinctures or infusions of antispasmodic and antimicrobial herbs, such as calendula, chamomile, licorice, garlic, sage, hyssop, peppermint, thyme, oregano, and elecampane. Don't use pau d'arco or goldenseal, as these herbs are too strong for babies and young children. Violet leaf can be an effective tonic for young children recovering from RSV.

Antioxidant herbs such as green tea and especially oregano can be effective in numerous circumstances. Oregano contains three to twenty times more antioxidants than other herbs, including garlic, and other fruits, including blueberries. According to a 2002 report, oregano (and its component rosmarinic acid) has "forty-two times more antioxidant activity than apples, thirty times more than potatoes, twelve times more than oranges and four times more than blueberries." [26]

Other antioxidant herbs, in order of strength, are dill, thyme, rosemary, and peppermint. Additionally, astragalus root and turmeric (also an anti-inflammatory useful for sore joints) have been shown to be effective in reducing the risk and severity of lung cancer.

The College of Pharmacy at the University of Illinois at Chicago relates a study describing the benefits of a Mediterranean diet along with the herbs rosemary, sage, parsley, and oregano in reducing the risk of lung cancer. [27] The University states that rosemary's phenolic diterpene, carnosol, has been evaluated for anticancer activity in prostate, breast, skin, and colon cancer as well as leukemia, and it may be effective against lung cancer as well.

Tier 2 specifics for the lower respiratory tract restore the lung's ability to circulate oxygen, absorb oxygen into the bloodstream, increase or decrease muscle contraction as needed, soothe, and either express (expectorant) or suppress (antitussive) coughs. Tier 3 corollary herbs soothe the throat, relieve headache or muscle ache from coughing, and ease nausea, among other adjunct symptoms.

Consider all the herbs described for the upper respiratory tract: garlic, licorice, mullein, yarrow, elderberry, sage, hyssop, peppermint, and thyme, as well as:

- **pleurisy root** (*Asclepias tuberosa*): commonly known as butterfly weed. The root of this lovely orange wildflower has long been used to ease lung congestion, suppress coughs, and reduce the

---

26 American Chemical Society (2002).

27 Johnson (2011).

inflammation associated with pleuritis and chronic coughing. This herb is anti-inflammatory, antimicrobial, anticatarrhal, and expectorant.

- **elecampane** (*Inula helenium*): a lovely tall flower that is easily cultivated. The root (and to a lesser extent the flower) contains sesquiterpene lactones and inulin. Elecampane is both mildly expectorant and strongly antitussive, acting as a powerful antispasmodic useful for chronic, hacking, and debilitating coughs, especially at night. Caution clients that they will feel a "squeeze" on their lungs as the herb takes effect, reducing their urge to cough.

- **horehound** *(Marrubium vulgare)*: horehound is another dual—or seemingly opposing—herb, combining both expectorant and antispasmodic actions. It is an extremely bitter herb that has traditionally been favored for unproductive coughs, dry hacking coughs, and whooping cough. Its expectorant ability is so strong it is contraindicated in pregnancy. Historically, horehound has been made into syrups, candies, and lozenges as it is too bitter to drink as a tea.

- **licorice** (*Glycyrrhiza glabra*): licorice combines triterpenes, flavonoids, coumarins, and polysaccharides into one of the most popular and reliable remedies in the herbal repertoire. It is a supreme demulcent, soothing mucous tissues and relieving irritation. (Caution: excessive use can cause retention of sodium and thus high blood pressure; avoid long-term use and use with care during pregnancy.)

- **coltsfoot** (*Tussilago farfara*): this lovely wildflower is high in the immune-supporting mineral zinc; its flowers are mucilaginous and its leaves are demulcent, expectorant, antitussive, and antispasmodic, useful in bronchitis and emphysema. Can be used in chronic pulmonary distress and asthma. Excellent nighttime remedy to suppress coughs to allow sleep, especially combined with mullein and elecampane.

- **wild cherry** *(Prunus serontina)*: the dried bark contains powerful glycosides that are antitussive, antispasmodic, expectorant, and astringent. Wild cherry bark is strongly antitussive and can be used for chronic conditions and acute infections. Historically used as a tonic for both respiratory and digestive support, and for convalescence; for those recovering from tuberculosis, pleurisy, pneumonia, and other diseases involving inflammation and bronchial debility.

- **yerba santa** *(Eriodictyon californicum)*: An evergreen native to the American Southwest, it was named "holy plant" by Spanish missionaries who witnessed the local Salinan, Ohlone, Miwok, Pomo, and Yokut tribes using the sticky leaves to treat lower respiratory diseases. Yerba santa is aromatic and used as a flavoring in foods, while infusions of the resinous leaves treat cough, fever, and indigestion. Leaves were smoked or chewed by locals; most yerba santa today is found in capsules.

- **eucalyptus** *(Eucalyptus globulus)*: the essential oil makes an effective steam-inhalation to relieve spasms of the lungs and act as an expectorant and antimicrobial. Avoid direct contact with eyes and nasal passages.

- **sage** *(Salvia officinalis)*: sage is a strong astringent and dries excessive catarrhal secretions in the lungs. Sometimes included in fragrant *kinnickkinnick* mixtures (along with mullein, uva ursi, and/or wild cherry bark).

- **white cedar** (*Thuja occidentalis*): white cedar (in the cypress family, not a true cedar) is antimicrobial and expectorant. Frequently used topically, the leaves (and even the sap) are high in essential oils and can be used—with discretion for respiratory illnesses, such as bronchitis—as a tea, liniment, or steam.

- **lobelia** (*Lobelia inflata*): also known as pukeweed or Indian tobacco is emetic and antispasmodic for the lungs and muscles. Used primarily in the treatment of asthma, whooping cough, and acute asthma. Not for long-term use.

- **skunk cabbage** (*Symplocarpus foetidus*): the roots are antispasmodic and were used in Native American medicine for coughs. This plant grows in bogs and swamps and smells terrible, but is unique in that it blooms very early (even in February) and puts out wonderfully large leaves (resembling comfrey) that keep the ground cool for other bog herbs, such as jewelweed. Caution: the fresh leaves are edible only when cooked.

- **khella** (*Ammi visnaga*): native to Europe, Asia, and North Africa, khella dilates bronchial vessels and relaxes smooth muscles, making it valuable for asthma.

Formulary for coughs generally depends on whether the cough is wet or dry. For wet coughs, tier 2 Specifics are astringents, with tier 3 corollary herbs addressing sore throat, bacterial infection, or sinus congestion. For dry coughs, tier 2 Specifics are demulcents, with tier 3 corollary herbs addressing sore throat, bacterial infection, or sore muscles from hacking coughs.

*Lower Respiratory Tract Formulas*

### A FORMULA FOR DRY, HACKING COUGH

> › 2 parts mullein
>
> › 1 part elecampane
>
> › 1 part lobelia
>
> › 1 part licorice

### A FORMULA FOR A WET, CROUPY COUGH

> › 2 parts elderberry
>
> › 1 part sage
>
> › 1 part coltsfoot
>
> › 1 part wild cherry

### A FORMULA FOR CHRONIC ASTHMA

> › 2 parts violet leaf
>
> › 1 part khella seed
>
> › 1 part mullein
>
> › 1 part pleurisy root

### A FORMULA TO SUPPORT HEALTHY LUNGS

> › 2 parts mullein
>
> › 1 part hyssop
>
> › 1 part sage
>
> › 1 part peppermint

Respiratory illness is a prime opportunity for using herbal remedies, and their use is well-documented and effective. Work with your clients and their support team to create formulas that both tone and nourish as well as treat the specific illness, using a variety of methods described here for a well-rounded approach to respiratory health.

# PART THREE

# Brain

Herbal medicine has a rich tradition of supporting the nerves. Physicians and scientists have been studying the nervous system since Aristotle, in the fourth century BCE, declared the nerves emanated from the heart. Galen determined that the nerves originated in the brain but he believed they were hollow in order that the person's spirit might flow through them; how else would a message be transmitted resulting in muscle movement or sensory perception? Much of Galen's writing in his *On the Natural Faculties* consists of bewildered questions about the presumed cavity in the hollow of the nerve, and he wonders at length how the nerve is nourished and what fluid must be inside. [28]

Despite the centuries of mystery surrounding the physics of the nervous system, herbalists have long observed direct effects from herbs on emotions and thought, and have cherished certain herbs for helping people stay calm, for instance, or relieving stress. Herbs ease anxiety, improve memory and are called nervous system herbs, nervine tonics, or cerebrotonic herbs. In this book, we will not address nootropics—controversial substances and plants that are used to improve memory, often induce a euphoric or even hallucinogenic feeling in the brain and are used recreationally or ceremonially (including caffeine, pharmaceutical drugs, and some herbs). Instead, while some of the herbs here can be classed as nootropics, the majority are used to physically support the cells in the brain and to

---

28    Stevenson, Daniel C. (2001).

strengthen our mental processes to such an extent that we perform at our peak mental level and feel emotionally healthy.

In chapter 6, we explore the functions of the nervous system and brain cells and look at nervine herbs and herbs for depression. In chapter 7 we will explore memory and mental clarity and Alzheimer's disease.

Refer to glossaries A, C, and D for details about the herbs and any contraindications.

## CHAPTER SIX

# The Brain and Nervous System

The nervous system is a complex and fascinating frontier, one of the final frontiers of human discovery and doubtless a mystery that may never be completely solved. For our purposes here, the central nervous system will be comprised of the brain and the brain stem, and the peripheral nervous system is the complex of nerves that allow us to sense what is in the world around us and to respond to these sensory observations with physiological and behavioral responses. All together, the nervous system allows us to think, reason, create, remember, and even to keep us safe, since the hormones and glands associated with quick action under threat are directed by the nervous system.

The largest (and heaviest) part of the brain is the cerebrum, the wrinkly grey matter that is the "bulk" of the brain. Commonly removed by Egyptian mummifiers as extraneous matter, the brain is now understood to be Grand Central Station for thought. The cerebrum, in particular, controls voluntary muscle movement as well as reasoning and deductive skills. Below the cerebrum lies the cerebellum, a smaller organ that controls body balance and the interplay between sensory organs and muscular activity. Beneath the cerebellum lies the brain stem that connects the brain to the spinal cord; the brain stem controls involuntary movements such as lung contraction and breath, heart muscle contraction, internal muscle contraction (of the stomach, the small intestine, and the large intestine), and other so-called reptilian activities that must be achieved without our consciously thinking about them.

Our brains have about a hundred billion nerve cells, or neurons, and more than a thousand trillion (10 to the 15th) connections between them. It's an incredibly complex (and miraculous) system that enables humans to send thought signals to affect actual movement and action. A neuron is part of a long chain of neurons. Each is separated by a synaptic cleft, the tiny space between neurons, the "yard between houses." This space is where much of the action happens—especially the action that can be affected by drugs and herbal medicines. At the very end of each presynaptic neuron sit little pouches full of neurotransmitters—the chemical messengers that stimulate the process of electrical transmission of information. Think of these as the kids in each house who want to go play in the yard. Their game is that they bunch up by the door, waiting for a special signal. When they get the signal, many of them run out the door and into the yard. The goal is to get to the other side—to the door of the next house—and send the signal along to the kids that are waiting at the next house.

There are many types of neurotransmitters that wait at the presynapse, including amino acids (glutamate), peptides (endorphines), and monoamines. Monoamines are responsible for attention, cognition, and emotion, and they include acetylcholine, serotonin, dopamine, noradrenaline, histamine, epinephrine, and norepinephrine. When an electrical signal comes down the axon (sending arm) of the neuron, its action potential stimulates the release of a particular neurotransmitter from its pouch. The neurotransmitter—say, the monoamine serotonin—expels from the pouch into the synaptic cleft. It then does one of several things:

1. It stays in the cleft, waiting.

2. It returns to the pouch in the presynaptic neuron.

3. It gets "eaten" by an enzyme (monoamine oxidase).

4. Or, it succeeds in traveling across the cleft to the next (postsynaptic) neuron. Here, it will either attach to a receptor and trigger an electrical impulse, or it will reach its final destination, such as a muscle, and trigger a muscle contraction.

The synaptic cleft is the place where herbs have a great potential for making a difference. One way they do this is by being a monoamine oxidase inhibitor.

## Monoamine Oxidase Inhibitor

If the neurotransmitters (monoamines) are the kids playing from one house to the next, the monoamine oxidase (MAO) is the kidnapper that snatches them out of the yard. MAO is the enzyme that breaks down neurotransmitters, taking them out of action and keeping them from reaching the next neuron. The signals (for happiness, joy, peace, serenity, muscle control, etc.) stop.

MAO-A breaks down serotonin, melatonin, epinephrine, norepinephrine, and dopamine. MAO-B breaks down dopamine, phenethylamine, and other trace amines.

The MAO-Inhibitor (MAOI) is the police officer that stops the kidnapper. MAOIs patrol the synapse and keep the oxidases from destroying neurotransmitters; as a result, the signals continue to the next neuron. The alkaloid harmaline is an example of a plant-based MAOI, particularly against MAO-A, which is why herbs with harmaline can be effective against depression. The herbs passionflower, Syrian rue, and nutmeg contain harmaline. Other apparent herbal MAOIs are turmeric, kava kava, and ayahuasca.

## Serotonin Reuptake Inhibitors

Another chemical that can stop the "game" of the neurotransmitters is one that "reuptakes" the neurotransmitter back into the neuron. If the monoamine is the kid running from one house through the yard to the next house, imagine the chemical as the grandma who yells, "Child! Get back in this house." The child reluctantly obeys, returning to the house; the monoamine is "reuptaken" into the neuron. This stops the progression of the electrical impulse moving across the synapse to the next neuron. (Monoamines can also return naturally to their "home" neuron.) The common result: depression.

But if you put a lock on the door, so to speak, the monoamine cannot return. This allows the neurotransmitter to stay in the synapse longer to fulfill its role and continue the electrical impulse. Herbs and drugs that "put the lock on" are called Selective Serotonin Reuptake Inhibitor (SSRI) because they inhibit the monoamine from returning. These likely include St. John's wort and licorice, though research on St. John's wort is contradictory. [29]

## Myelin Sheath Protectors

Finally, some herbs help support the production of the myelin sheath, which is the fatty tissue that surrounds the neuron's axon, promoting the transmission of the electrical information. The myelin sheath insulates the axon in intervals, keeping the sodium and potassium from "leaking" out of the axon and allowing the action potential to jump from one Node of Ranvier (action site between the sheaths) to the next, increasing the rate of

---

29   Wheatley, David (2002).

transmission. In other words, the better the myelin sheath, the faster the signals move from the brain to the body.

A lack of myelin sheath is the basis of multiple sclerosis (MS), a disease in which the body's own immune system actually attacks and dismantles the sheath around the neuron in the central nervous system, causing scar tissue to develop and disrupting muscle control, vision, speech, and voluntary movement. Amyotrophic lateral sclerosis (ALS), also called Lou Gehrig's disease, occurs when the nerve cells die completely, causing an atrophy of the muscles. Certain herbs are being researched for their potential role in protecting the myelin sheath and easing symptoms associated with MS and ALS. Cinnamate, a compound found in cinnamon, storax (*Liquidamber orientalis* or benzoic resin), and shea butter, appears to block lactate transport, which can ease muscle fatigue for symptomatic relief.

More directly, turmeric may be of assistance in protecting the myelin sheath. In 2002, the *Journal of Immunology* reported the ability of curcumin, the so-called "active" ingredient in turmeric root, to substantially reduce the inflammatory demyelination response in mice afflicted with EAE, the mouse version of multiple sclerosis. [30] More recently, curcumin is the focus of researchers at Vanderbilt University who recognize the plant's ability to destroy the beta-amyloid plaques of Alzheimer's disease but who have been stymied by curcumin's inability to cross the blood-brain barrier. [31] To overcome this obstacle, Vanderbilt and Japanese researchers developed a curcumin analog that can be made into an aerosol and inhaled, bypassing the blood-brain barrier. Their studies in mice suggest that aerosol applications might be helpful for humans suffering with either Alzheimer's, MS, and related diseases of myelin sheath degeneration.

---

30   Natarajan C., and John Bright (2002).

31   Jumbo-Lucioni, Patricia (2015).

## Parkinson's Disease

A healthy supply of dopamine supports balance, muscle control, impulse control, attention, wakefulness and energy, and assertiveness. Too little leads to anxiety, frustration, violence, and muscle tremors. It also leads to Parkinson's disease. In PD, the neurons that produce dopamine die off or stop their use of dopamine, affecting the movement of the hands and legs and even speaking and swallowing. Ashwagandha, turmeric, astragalus, and codonopsis warrant more study for their effects on Parkinson's disease; the following herbs are also worth mentioning:

- **velvet bean** (*Mucuna pruriens*): a study of the powdered bean of this vine lists velvet bean as a "natural source of L-dopa" and reports that individuals in the trial experienced rapid onset of anti-spasmodic action and a longer interval between needed doses. [32]

- **griffonia** (*Griffonia simplicifolia*): this plant's seeds yield 5-Hydroxy-L-tryptophan (5-HTP), which is extracted in laboratories from this woody shrub native to West-Central Africa. The chemical extract has numerous studies attributing to it activity against both Parkinson's and depression. [33]

- **corydalis** (*Corydalis cava*): more traditionally used as a sedative, hypnotic, and analgesic, the roots of this herb are gaining popularity for use in Parkinson's disease, as its complex alkaloids show antispasmodic activity. [34] Some herbalists use the herb to ease spasms and pain in the pelvis, especially for women with chronic pelvic pain (CPP). [35]

---

32   Katzenschlager, Evans, and Manson (2004).

33   Thompson Healthcare Inc. (2007).

34   Ibid. 232.

35   Romm, Aviva (2010), 247.

## Parkinson's Disease Formulas
### A FORMULA FOR MUSCLE SPASMS IN PARKINSON'S

> › 2 parts turmeric
>
> › 1 part astragalus
>
> › 1 part velvet bean
>
> › 1 part St. John's wort

## Calming and Nervine Herbs

Another neurotransmitter is noradrenaline. This stress hormone is produced by the sympathetic neurons of the heart and stimulates myocardial contractions. It also stimulates stress-related behavioral and physiological responses to danger, which can result in increased heart rate, shallow breathing, increased dispersal of glucose throughout the body, increased dispersal of blood to skeletal muscles and constriction of skeletal muscles, dilation of pupils, and increased blood flow to the brain. These are commonly called the fight-or-flight responses and are essential to the survival of an organism under pressure or attack.

Many plants that contain chemicals that produce exactly the opposite effect, calming the body, relaxing the muscles, easing the breathing, calming the mind—and they've been used traditionally to reverse this process in acute situations and to prevent it from happening in chronic-stress situations. Consider:

- **motherwort** (*Leonurus cardiaca*): As its name suggests, heart of the lion has been used as a cardiotonic to strengthen the heart. This bitter-tasting herb is also a spasmolytic to reduce the angry effects of tight, tense muscles. The leaves contain the alkaloid leonurine, a vasodilator that allows greater flow of blood through the vessels and eases the pressure on the heart, reducing blood pressure. This lessens pressure on the peripheral nervous system, as well, relieving feelings of frustration, tension, and panic. Motherwort has the potential to mitigate or reverse the effects of noradrenaline.

- **skullcap** (*Scutellaria lateriflora*): Long appreciated as a nervine tonic, skullcap is used for anxiety, headache, and insomnia—all effects of the production of noradrenaline from acute or chronic stress. The use of skullcap has been contested, however, by herbalists such as Varro Tyler, who point to studies in which there was no relief noticed for the use of the herb. Other studies have shown a benefit and a distinct difference between American skullcap (*S. lateriflora*) and Chinese skullcap (*S. baicalensis*), with American skullcap leaf acting as a sedative and nervine tonic, and Chinese skullcap root acting as an antispasmodic and anti-inflammatory, especially useful for headaches. It may also have some anti-cancer properties. Both forms of skullcap have been subject to dishonest substitution usually with germander (*Teucrium chamaedrys*), a hepatotoxic.

- **passionflower** (*Passiflora incarnata*): traditionally for anxiety, insomnia, seizures, and hysteria. It is believed to work by increasing GABA levels in the brain, and since gamma aminobutyric acid is the primary inhibitory or sedating neurotransmitter, increasing GABA lowers the effects of noradrenaline, promotes relaxation, and sedates an over-stimulated mind and body.

### Calming and Nervine Formulas
#### A FORMULA FOR CHRONIC STRESS (WARMING)
> › 2 parts rhodiola
> › 1 part licorice
> › 1 part cinnamon
> › 1 part holy basil

### A FORMULA FOR CHRONIC STRESS (COOLING)

> › 2 parts eleuthero
> › 1 part lemon balm
> › 1 part motherwort
> › 1 part licorice

### A FORMULA FOR EXCITATORY ANXIETY

> › 2 parts ashwagandha
> › 1 part motherwort
> › 1 part passionflower or St. John's wort
> › 1 part chamomile

## *Depression, Post-Traumatic Stress Disorder, and Post-Partum Depression*

Illnesses associated with mild, moderate, and severe depression include post-traumatic stress disorder (PTSD), post-partum depression (PPD), and, of course, depression, among others. These conditions vary widely in their cause (PTSD seems to be experience-related and also injury-related while PPD appears hormonally driven), though they share many of the same symptoms: fatigue, loss of will to act, confusion, sadness, bleakness, and in many cases a tendency toward violence against self or others.

Working in tandem with counselors and other healing arts professionals, consider the following herbs in a formula that includes antidepressants and nervine tonics and perhaps cardiotonics and digestive aids:

- **lemon balm** (*Melissa officinalis*): mildly sedative, lemon balm is carminative and spasmolytic as appreciated in digestion. It is also antiviral and is approved by the Commission E for nervousness and insomnia. [36] Lemon balm is ideal for conditions where sadness, grief, and depression interfere with clarity of thought.

---

36   American Botanical Council (1990).

- **passionflower** (*Passiflora incarnata*): the leaves, and to a lesser extent the flowers, contain alkaloids and other compounds that bind to the same areas of the brain influenced by GABA, acting to calm the nervous system; passionflower is anxiolytic and in some people is sedative. Contraindicated in pregnancy.

- **rhodiola** (*Rhodiola rosea*): this flavonoid-rich, Northern Hemisphere wildflower has a pronounced effect on the central nervous system. It is considered an adaptogen and anxiolytic and has been the subject of numerous clinical and laboratory studies. The root has demonstrated significant anti-fatigue and endurance effects, despite the plant's lack of caffeine, and it is an effective herb to treat depression that is brought about by chronic fatigue, overwork, excessive physical activity, and overexertion. [37] It is contraindicated in people with bipolar disorder, especially those with a high-manic tendency.

- **St. John's wort** (*Hypericum perforatum*): St. John's Wort apparently works in part because of its "reuptake" effect on the monoamine neurotransmitter serotonin. Serotonin is primarily found in the gastrointestinal tract, where it helps manage gut muscle movements. But a small part of the human body's serotonin is found in the central nervous system where it regulates mood, appetite, cognitive functions, such as memory and learning, and desire for or ability to sleep. (Serotonin also gets into the bloodstream and helps with the clotting factor of platelets.) St. John's wort has been studied extensively as an antidepressant and shows activity as a GABA binder and MAOI. The herb apparently increases the liver's ability to metabolize certain chemicals, making

---

37  Robertsdottir (2013), 296.

it contraindicated in clients already taking other MAOIs, antico-agulants, or other prescription medications. [38]

## Depression, Post-Traumatic Stress Disorder, and Post-Partum Depression Formulas

### A FORMULA FOR MILD, OCCASIONAL DEPRESSION

› 2 parts oats milky tops

› 1 part St. John's wort

› 1 part lavender

› 1 part holy basil

### A FORMULA FOR MILD, CHRONIC DEPRESSION

› 2 parts rhodiola

› 2 parts lemon balm

› 1 part peppermint

› 1 part passionflower

### A FORMULA FOR POST-TRAUMATIC STRESS DISORDER (PTSD)

› 2 parts linden

› 1 part motherwort

› 1 part eleuthero

› 1 part turmeric

### A FORMULA FOR POST-TRAUMATIC STRESS DISORDER (PTSD)

› 2 parts eleuthero

› 1 part motherwort

---

38   Romm (2010), 544.

> 1 part St. John's wort

> 1 part oats

## A FORMULA FOR POST-PARTUM DEPRESSION (PPD)

> 2 parts motherwort

> 2 parts oats

> 1 part eleuthero

> 1 part yellow dock

> 1 part lemon balm

## ANOTHER FORMULA FOR POST-PARTUM DEPRESSION (PPD)

> 2 parts holy basil (tulsi)

> 1 part lemon balm

> 1 part angelica

> 1 part black cohosh

## A FORMULA FOR MILD DEPRESSION

> 2 parts St. John's wort

> 2 parts lemon balm

> 2 parts oats milky tops

> 1 part eleuthero

## A FORMULA FOR MILD DEPRESSION WITH NO DESIRE TO EAT

> 2 parts motherwort

> 1 part chamomile

> 1 part holy basil

> 1 part nettle

## ADD/ADHD

The symptom complexes of attention deficit disorder (ADD) and attention deficit hyperactivity disorder (ADHD) are easy to spot but are of indeterminate origin. No one has been able to pinpoint one particular cause of ADD or ADHD, though genetics, environmental factors, diet, and neurological factors have all been implicated, and due to this complexity and the rampant diagnoses in the United States in recent years, a complete discussion of ADD/ADHD is beyond the scope of this book. However, many herbs used both traditionally and clinically are relevant for the healing arts practitioner interested in introducing herbs into a therapeutic practice.

Dr. Tieraona Low Dog mentions "disorder of the … dopamine systems" as a possible cause and suggests herbs such as lemon balm that affect the limbic-hippocampal area of the brain [39]; other ideas suggest the disorders stem from brain circuit abnormalities. The hippocampus is tentatively identified as an organ responsible for helping people maintain both short-term and long-term memory, as it provides the "glue" that helps memories stick, and lemon balm directly affects it:

- **lemon balm** (*Melissa officinale*): helpful in cases of memory loss, mental clarity and ADD/ADHD, this fragrant herb affects the limbic-hippocampal area of the brain and its official uses are for nervousness and insomnia. It strengthens mental processes and is a favorite of test-takers and students, helping the hippocampus "sift" through what memories need glue and which ones don't, allowing a child with ADD/ADHD to let go of excessive, irrelevant, or confusing stimuli. Lemon balm is antidepressant and is a prime tier 1 tonic for stress, tension or anxiety and a tier 2 specific for focus in ADD/ADHD.

---

39  Low Dog (1997).

### *ADD/ADHD Formulas*
#### A FORMULA FOR ADD, FOR FOCUS

› 2 parts lemon balm

› 1 part eleuthero

› 1 part ginkgo

› 1 part peppermint

#### A FORMULA FOR ADD/ADHD

› 2 parts lemon balm

› 1 part ashwagandha

› 1 part oats milky tops

› 1 part vervain

Collaborating with a client's primary care providers, counselors, family, and other support team members is the best way to support his or her mental health in both acute and chronic conditions. Herbs can play a vital role in the improvement of these conditions and the nourishment of the brain and nervous system as a whole.

# CHAPTER SEVEN

# Memory and Cognitive Thought

Herbalism plays a starring role in therapies that strengthen cognition and memory, and research shows its efficacy in helping people with dementia recover their cognitive abilities and improve their quality of life—which is what true herbalism is all about: improving a person's physical and mental function such that a person feels loved, capable, confident, productive, and independent—this is the true nature of using healing plants. In this chapter, we will focus on true mental processes and the illnesses that can affect cerebral function, memory, clarity of thought, and mental acuity. Some of the herbal actions required when dealing with these issues are:

- Nervine tonics to support the central nervous system and assist with coping mechanisms

- Cerebrotonics to bring blood flow to the brain and support cerebral function

- Adaptogens to support the nervous system as it adapts and reacts to stress

- Vasodilators to increase blood flow to the brain and the periphery

- Bitters and lymphatics to clear out the digestive system and improve the flow of fluids, relieving "sluggish" digestion

## Memory and Mental Clarity

Humans have long been fascinated with memory; how is it we can revisualize or recall something that happened in the past? Why do we remember certain events but not others? How can cultures have what scientists call "collective" memories, or what Carl Jung called the "collective unconscious"? How do memories affect our emotions, or even our physical health?

The study of memory is termed cognitive neuroscience, and it is a vast and complex interdisciplinary study of thought, emotion, society, and physics. Many scientists and psychologists look to the synapses between neural cells that carry electrical impulses, and they study the hippocampus and other prefrontal lobe structures of the brain. For herbalists, a holistic treatment will focus on the individual's social needs, physical abilities, diet, and herbs that address blood flow to or inflammation in the brain. Sprinkled throughout this will be tonics that support, calm, or stimulate the various systems of the body—even seemingly unconnected systems such as the circulatory and the digestive.

Mental fog, memory loss, and mental disability (acute and chronic) can be brought on by any number of disparate factors in males and females of any age: menopause and hormone changes in both women and men; sports injury or other injury involving head trauma; stroke; ischemia (restriction of blood supply to a particular area of the body); drug overdose; and infection. A number of herbs are tier 2 Specifics for mental clarity, gaining clarity of thought during menopause when the brain feels "foggy," or enhancing the well-being of the mind:

- **lemon balm** (*Melissa officinalis*): as mentioned, lemon balm is commonly used as a safe tier 1 nervine tonic. Used to calm, soothe, and tone the central nervous system. It provides an elevated feeling of well-being and even joy and is called a "gladdening herb." It is also a favorite of test-takers and is widely used for ADD/ADHD to provide focus and the ability to block out background stimuli.

- **cocoa** (*Theobroma cacao*): though processed chocolate contains sweeteners and flavorings, cacao itself is high in a variety of alkaloids including theobromine, caffeine, and phenethylamine that may stimulate serotonin levels. It's widely known to jump-start the mood and temporarily improve mental clarity. Use sparingly as a tier 3 or 4 herb.

- **gotu kola** (*Centella asiatica*): an edible herb that can easily be grown in the garden, gotu kola is an anxiolytic and an adaptogen, widely appreciated for anxiety and stress as well as mental clarity and brain function.[40] It is a tier 1 tonic and is used as a cerebral tonic and circulatory stimulant directing blood flow to the brain much like ginkgo.

- **rosemary** (*Rosmarinus officinalis*): a strong circulatory stimulant, rosemary is much stronger than gotu kola and should be used with caution internally, and only short term. The essential oils in rosemary make it an exceptional vulnerary externally and their inhalation is being studied as a new treatment for Alzheimer's disease (see page 142).

---

40   McIntyre (2013).

- **ginger** (*Zingiber officinale*): an exotic spice used as a food, ginger is a pleasant tasting rhizome that stimulates blood flow both internally and externally. It is an aromatic digestive aid useful for nausea, and it tends to clear the mind and offer sharper thinking. It is gaining widespread use as an anxiolytic and is believed to play a role in serotonin reuptake.

- **ginkgo** (*Ginkgo biloba*): the leaves of this ancient tree are traditionally used to enhance memory. Long used in folk medicine, ginkgo has undergone extensive clinical research with varying results. Its memory effects may stem from its ability to inhibit the reuptake of norepinephrine. A vasodilator, ginkgo can be considered at any tier in a formula for memory and cognitive thought.

- **schisandra** (*Schisandra chinensis*): a nourishing and strengthening tier 1 tonic for many systems of the body, this herb is used in traditional Chinese medicine and throughout Eastern cultures as an adaptogen. [41]

- **peppermint** (*Mentha piperita*): commonly used to relieve sinus congestion and strengthen capillary function as a mild cardiovascular stimulant, peppermint (generally stronger than spearmint) is useful for mental clarity formulas because it boosts blood flow around the body. Use peppermint in tier 2, 3, or 4.

- **wild sarsaparilla** (*Aralia nudicaulis*): not to be confused with sarsaparilla (*Smilax*), the slender running roots of this North American wildflower provide, especially in tincture form, a boost of energy without caffeine. Used for stamina and endurance, this is a tier 3 or 4 herb for mental acuity and memory.

---

41   Winston (2013).

- **oats** (*Avena sativa*): a nourishing tier 1 tonic for the entire body, especially for the central nervous system. Mineral-rich and sustaining.

- **linden** (*Tilia europa* or *T. cordata*): also call lime blossom or basswood, this nervine tonic is traditionally used to relieve hysteria and support cardiovascular health. Linden is used in formulas for mental clarity as a tier 1 tonic or a tier 4 vehicle.

- **hawthorn** (*Cretaegous* spp.): the leaves, berries and flowers act as cardiotonics, vasodilators, and nervine tonics and they can be used in mental clarity formulas as tier 1 or tier 3. Particularly valuable for cognitive and cerebral function since the risk factors for dementia are nearly the same as the risk factors for cardiac illness.

## Herbalism for the Elderly

Since memory issues are often (but not always) associated with growing older, the healing arts practitioner will need to consider the age of the client. Dementia, of which Alzheimer's disease is a type, can affect anyone beginning around the average age of sixty-five. (Dementia before this age is called "early onset dementia.") Be sure, when working with elderly clients, to address their quality of life first: Are they enjoying their current relationships? Are they continuing to develop new relationships, new dynamics? Everyone, regardless of age, should be continually piquing their curiosity and expanding their awareness; otherwise life is dull and the mind cannot reach its highest imaginative and joyful potential.

Aging men and women typically experience changes (weakening) of the bones and skin; they develop gray hair, weakening eyesight, cardio issues (stiffening of arteries), and a lower bodily mineral content. But older people have qualities that younger people can envy: they possess incredible life skills that can only come from experience, they have passed through all the phases of life; and they can advise and counsel in politics, reform, business, health, and family. Herbal heritage celebrates aging and recognizes that our elderly men and women symbolize valuable qualities desperately needed by our contemporary cultures. This stage of life is, ideally, one of wonder, reflection, and sharing.

## Dementia and Alzheimer's Disease

There are a number of different types of dementia, which include Alzheimer's disease and senility. Alzheimer's disease typically develops beginning about age sixty-five and is the sixth leading cause of death in the United States. After noticeable onset, complications cause physical deterioration so that life expectancy is eight years. [42] In Alzheimer's, the brain produces plaques made of beta-amyloid, a normal protein "clipped" off from its parent protein that becomes problematic. The brain also produces tangles made of tau proteins that collapse and twist into tangled knots, destroying the normal pathways of neurons. The brain also shows inflammation, oxidative change, and (frequently) metal toxicity.

While genetics are strongly implicated (scientists have discovered a single gene (ApoE4) that greatly increases the risk of developing Alzheimer's), [43] there seem to be other causes as well: stroke, Parkinson's disease, HIV/AIDS, Huntington's disease, and traumatic brain injury can lead to the brain damage that causes dementia. Even being an alcoholic has been shown to increase the risk of developing dementia significantly, and emotional or cognitive states, such as depression, and physical diseases such as diabetes or thyroid dysfunction can impede memory loss and learning patterns. Certain medications can lead to memory impairment, such as sedatives and sleeping pills, painkillers, and a stomach medication called

---

42   Alzheimer's Association (2016).

43   National Institute on Aging (2016).

cimetidine, among others. Alarmingly, Alzheimer's disease is increasingly being linked to diabetes.

Research published in the *Journal of Diabetes Science and Technology* concluded that AD is actually type 3 diabetes that targets the brain.[44] We are beginning to understand the way the brain processes insulin and its role in dementia, particularly Alzheimer's. Insulin is a peptide, a small protein, produced in the pancreas in response to glucose (the body and brain's main fuel). Glucose needs insulin to be transported into cells. Just like other cells of the body, neurons need insulin to allow the glucose in so they can properly function (for muscle movement as well as memory, attention, and thinking). When insulin is not working properly, glucose cannot get into cells. It builds up outside the cells and stays in the blood and initiates "insulin resistance." The brain realizes the cells aren't getting glucose so it produces even more insulin. The pancreas can't keep up with the amount of insulin the body thinks it needs; it goes into overdrive and quickly becomes deficient. Meanwhile, glucose builds up to dangerous levels in the blood. Over time, this leads to diabetes. Cellular starvation and high blood glucose levels lead to inflammation in the body—and possibly to beta-amyloid accumulation in the brain.

### Herbal Therapy

Though herbal medicine does not have a long tradition treating Alzheimer's disease, since it was only identified and named in 1906, we do have substantial experience supporting mental clarity and health and increasing cognitive awareness and cerebral function.

Interestingly, most of the risk factors that lead to cardiac illnesses are the same factors that lead to dementia; herbalists can use this information by understanding that the same strategies that keep the heart healthy will

---

44   Monte and Wands (2008).

also be of great benefit in keeping the mind healthy. The cardiac guidelines in chapter 4 are relevant to cerebral health and mental clarity.

In addition to gotu kola and hawthorn, consider:

- **ginkgo** (*Ginkgo biloba*): may delay the deterioration of neural cells presumably by increasing oxygen to those cells as a vasodilator. Ginkgo contains the flavonoid quercetin, a potent free radical scavenger, and it tends to improve patients with senile macular degeneration.

- **ginseng** (*Panax ginseng*): In animal studies (in mice), ginseng alcohol extracts stimulated insulin release and decreased serum levels of glucose. These studies also looked at ginseng berry (in addition to the root) and found positive anti-diabetes effects. [45]

- **bitter melon** (*Momordica charantia*): its hypoglycemic effects demonstrated in cell culture, animal models, and human studies make it particularly valuable in Alzheimer's studies since Alzheimer's is being called type 3 diabetes. In one study, bitter melon "improved glucose tolerance in type 2 diabetics by preventing sugar from being absorbed into the intestines." Bitter melon increased insulin products and the mass of beta cells in the pancreas. [46]

- **coptis chenensis** (*Huang lian*): decreased fasting blood glucose levels in diabetic rats in studies. [47] Other herbs that contain the alkaloid berberine, believed to be the active compound in coptis, include Oregon grape and goldenseal, making them all the subjects of clinical research for Alzheimer's therapy.

---

45   Hui, Tang, and Liang W Go (2009).

46   Ibid.

47   Hui, Tang, and Liang W Go (2009).

- **bacopa** (*Bacopa monnieri*): also called Brahmi, but not to be confused with gotu kola. Bacopa is a low-growing succulent that thrives in wet conditions. In lab studies, bacopa extract displayed antioxidant polyphenols that reduced divalent metals, decreased the formation of lipid peroxides, and reduced beta-amyloid plaques in the brains of Alzheimer's stricken test animals.

- **cubeb** (*Piper cubeba*): also called java pepper, this Indonesian shrub produces tiny berries high in essential oils and is used as an aromatic for digestive complains, bronchial ailments, and poor memory.

- **rhodiola** (*Rhodiola rosea*): the roots of this cold-loving sedum-like Arctic herb are being studied for their beneficial effects on mental clarity. The rhizomes showed monoamine oxidase inhibition (A & B) activity in research trials, specifically demonstrating antidepression potential by inhibiting MOA-A and senile dementia potential by inhibiting MOA-B. [48] Long a favorite of Asian and European folk medicine, rhodiola is a key player in the efforts to stem progressive dementia and cognitive impairment.

- **rosemary** (*Rosmarinus officinalis*) high in flavonoids, di-and tri-terpenes, and volatile oils, rosemary is the herb Shakespeare's Ophelia described as the herb for memory. Commonly used topically as an antiseptic, rosemary can be taken internally in small amounts for short periods of time for antimicrobial and antiviral purposes. Recent studies have confirmed rosemary's tumor-inhibiting effects. Like ginkgo, it is a circulatory stimulant and vasodilatory to the periphery and brain, used traditionally to relieve headaches and dizziness." Do not use during pregnancy.

---

48   Dierman, Marston, and Bravo (2009).

- **periwinkle** (*Vinca minor*): used in European folk medicine to treat cognitive impairment and memory loss, periwinkle contains alkaloids that make it both effective and potentially toxic. Known to stimulate blood flow to the brain and even assist with metabolism in the brain itself, periwinkle is used to produce vinpocetine and the vinca-based prescription drug Cavinton for cerebrovascular disorders and age-related memory dysfunction.[49] Other beneficial alkaloids from periwinkle include vinblastine and vincristine, which are widely regarded as strong chemotherapeutic agents with anticancer potential.

- **cinnamon** (*Cinnamomum* spp.): a growing body of research supports cinnamon as a treatment for dementia, with direct impact on beta-amyloid plaques as well as direct influence on insulin levels and diabetes control.[50]

- **turmeric** (*Curcuma longa*): Turmeric and its chemical curcumin have proven strongly therapeutic for the brain and the neural cells, assisting with neurotransmitter movement, the myelin sheath, and the reduction and possible prevention of the beta-amyloid plaques of Alzheimer's. Turmeric is recognized by the National Cancer Institute as an anticarcinogen, both *in-vitro* and *in-vivo*.[51] A study at UCLA found curcumin may help the immune system's macrophages clear beta amyloid accumulation, and, the study found that curcumin improves the creation of the fatty myelin sheath surrounding nerve cells, an extraordinary process by glial cells called myelogenesis.[52]

---

49  Thompson Healthcare Inc. (2007).

50  Frydman-Marom, Levin, and Farfara (2011).

51  Shrikant and Palanivelu (2008).

52  Zhang, et al. (2006).

## Dementia and Alzheimer's Disease Formulas

### A FORMULA FOR EARLY-ONSET ALZHEIMER'S DISEASE

› 2 parts hawthorn

› 2 parts turmeric

› 1 part cinnamon

› 1 part ginkgo

### A FORMULA FOR DEMENTIA WITH IRRITABILITY

› 2 parts lemon balm

› 1 part rhodiola

› 1 part rosemary

› 1 part rose

### A FORMULA FOR POSSIBLE DEMENTIA PREVENTION

› 2 parts turmeric

› 1 part cinnamon

› 1 part bacopa

› 1 part peppermint

› ½ part black pepper

The more we learn about the intricate processes of the brain, and especially how brain health is connected to other organs and systems of the body (such as the endocrine and the complex insulin-regulating systems), the more we will appreciate the contribution herbs have to offer. The use of herbs in formulas, in collaboration with other healing arts modalities, is full of promise.

# PART FOUR

# Immune System, Skin, and First Aid

The healing arts practitioner has a wealth of herbal knowledge to pull from in supporting the immune system and healing the skin. Long a vague concept, immunity is now better understood and the role of herbal medicines is widely accepted as effective and safe. Use the following formulas and guidelines to craft both preventive and curative remedies and to create skin and first aid medicines that will prove useful in a wide variety of settings.

# CHAPTER EIGHT

# The Immune System

Of all the body's mysteries, the immune system seems to be one of the most recent to be examined with any real depth of understanding. Very complex and seemingly delicate, the immune system comprises a myriad of systems within the body organized to keep us healthy: the lymph system, the circulatory system, the skin (integumentary system), the liver (its own mystery), and to some degree the glandular system. All of these interact in a very precise and efficient way to keep out debris and foreign organisms, to kill invading parasites and pathogens, and to restore vitality after an illness.

A complete understanding of immunity will involve a detailed education in lymphocytes, immunological memory, autoimmunity, interferon production, inflammation, and even cancerous tumors, all of which are beyond the scope of this book. But plant remedies support the function of the immune system and also kill pathogens, and immune-support herbs feature in our formulas. The immune system consists of two basic parts:

the innate system, which provides a general response to a new infection, and the adaptive system, which provides a specific response to a previously identified pathogen. The innate or general system uses phagocytes, neutrophils, macrophages, and dendritic cells to accomplish its goals. The adaptive system uses antibodies and is the result of "acquired immunity." In the adaptive system, various specialized proteins, cells, and organs detect other cells, proteins, and enzymes, and they distinguish these from "normal" inhabitants of the body, create a "memory" of this attacker, employ white cells to abolish the attacker, and send a letter of reference to the brain to record the memory and create "memory cells" so when this attacker comes again, the entire immune defense will immediately recognize it and act. But autoimmune diseases, such as AIDS, wreak havoc with this system by intercepting that letter to the brain and by deceiving the proteins and cells into thinking normal cells are the attackers. What causes autoimmune diseases? Viruses and bacteria can. Also pharmaceutical and other drugs can interfere with the immune process. Even genetics can play a role in whether the immune system succeeds or suffers. Previously mysterious diseases have now been classified as autoimmune diseases, such as diabetes mellitus type 1, lupus, and rheumatoid arthritis, for example.

A number of cells are important in this system:

- **leukocytes:** white blood cells present in all tissue, including the brain, spinal cord, central nervous system, blood, and lymphatic system. Special leukocytes include neutrophils, eosinophils, basophils, lymphocytes, and monocytes. Doctors check for an elevated level of leukocytes in the blood that may indicate infection or disease.

- **lymphocytes:** a type of white blood cell specific to lymph fluid. Three types are primary: NK, T, and B cells.

- **NK cells:** a type of lymphocyte that supports innate or general immune response by identifying virus-infected cells and destroying them.

- **T cells (thymus cell) and B cells (bone-marrow cells):** lymphocytes that support the adaptive immune response by identifying invaders, producing antibodies, and promoting "memory cells" so the organism remembers the invader for future attacks.

- **cytokines:** complex proteins that trigger responses from other cells' receptors, acting as a communication service. These are messengers of the immune system.

Additionally, there are two fascinating mechanisms by which herbs and pharmaceuticals influence the immune system:

1. **Toll-Like Receptors.** Certain proteins stay on the outside of our immune system cells and "scan" for bacteria, fungi, etc. They recognize patterns (pathogen-associated molecular patterns, or PAMPs) that are produced by the pathogens. Certain herbs (such as astragalus, wild yam, and echinacea) contain polysaccharides that apparently mimic these patterns, stimulating an immune response. [53]

2. **Efflux Pump Inhibitor.** Bacteria can live on the outside of cells, especially around wounds. They produce cytotoxins which are delivered to the interior of the cell through a pump, wounding or killing the cell. Certain herbs (including turmeric, ginseng, kava, barberry, goldenseal (an at-risk plant), milk thistle, and mushrooms such as reishi contain chemicals that inhibit this pump, shutting down the bacteria's pathway into the cell and making the bacteria inert. [54]

---

53  Clare (2012).

54  Ibid.

# Herbal Actions for the Immune System

When referring to the immune system, Americans speak in war terms: we say we are "fighting" a cold, our medicines are "attacking" germs, or we have achieved "victory" over illness. While in some regard our body's cells and systems are indeed protecting us from "invading" pathogens, it would be just as easy to use housecleaning terms such as sweeping, cleaning, and disinfecting. Health is not so much a matter of destroying the other camp but maintaining a cycle. Our chemistry is constantly adapting, changing, and morphing because we live in a natural and complex environment.

Nevertheless, when we discuss immunity, we use words such as antiviral, antibacterial, antiparasitic (also called vermifuge), antifungal, and anti-inflammatory. Immune support involves both killing pathogens and, if we can, supporting the formation and function of neurophils, eosinophils, monocytes, and lymphocytes (commonly called white blood cells) including B-cells and T-cells. We strive to maintain a balance so that unhealthy bacteria don't over-colonize and kill off the "good" bacteria, so that we don't succumb to every bacteria with which we come in contact.

First we'll explore basic antibacterial, antiparasitic, and antiviral herbs, then we'll feature plants that provide long-term support to maintain a strong immune system.

## Bacteria and Antibacterial Herbs

These are the herbs believed through heritage or proven clinically to have the capacity to either kill pathogens directly or to support the body's efforts to kill them. Often used topically, many of these herbs are appropriate for internal bactericide, though care must be used in taking them internally because their potency can damage the liver and other organs. Small doses are used, and many of these herbs are used "whole," though their powerful essential oils can be isolated and diluted in salves, liniments, and compresses. Essential oils are rarely used internally and such use is not encouraged in this book.

- **oregano, thyme, rosemary, lavender, sage:** all of Mediterranean origin, these can be used as health-promoting foods in the diet as well as in more concentrated forms such as teas, capsules, tablets, compresses, poultices, liniments, syrups, and tinctures. These herbs are frequently used for bacterial infections of the skin (topical infections), wounds, and infections of the soft tissues of the sinuses, mouth, and digestive tract.

- **calendula** *(Calendula officinalis)*: a strong antimicrobial, antifungal, and emollient, calendula is an excellent choice for soothing inflammation and infection of the skin and soft tissues. Frequently used in formulas for treating eczema, psoriasis, and *Candida albicans*. Many herbalists find it effective for regulating abnormal cells such as those found in cervical dysplasia, topical skin tumors, and abscessed wounds.

- **elecampane** *(Inula helenium)*: the root is used in formulas for bronchial infection. One of the strongest cough suppressants in the herbal repertoire, excellent for a nagging cough. It is a powerful muscle relaxant and works quickly on bronchial spasms and can be effective for other spastic muscles.

- **goldenseal** *(Hydrastis canadensis)* and Oregon grape root *(Mahonia* spp): Both on the United Plant Savers Lists (see Glossary E). Goldenseal is an effective antibacterial and astringent, ideal for infections involving excess mucus or fluid production, pus-filled infections, diarrhea, bowel infections, and weepy open sores.

- **clove oil, eucalyptus oil, tea tree oil:** These three are powerful antiseptics, rarely used internally and prized for their ability to control and eradicate infection on the skin. Tea tree oil derives from the *Melaleuca* tree and is comprised of its inner bark and the essential oils distilled from that bark. Tea tree has gained a reputation as an all-natural fungicide and bactericide, being used to treat (mostly) topical infections. Use these diluted on the skin and do not ingest the essential oils.

- **licorice** (*Glycyrrhiza glabra*): A member of the legume family, licorice is so named because "glyc" refers to sugar and "rhiza" refers to the rhizome or root. Licorice is a bronchial antispasmodic and antitussive, lessening cough and soothing inflamed lung tissues. Its glycerrhizic acid is known to boost interferon production, alerting immune function when bacteria and viruses enter the body. In Oriental medicine, licorice counteracts chronic viral hepatitis, and in Western herbalism it treats the viral ulcer-forming *Helicobacter pylori* and soothes stomach and duodenal ulcers. Overuse of licorice can raise blood pressure.

### Fungi and Antifungal Herbs

Antifungal herbs are those that directly kill fungal infections or aid the body in attacking fungal pathogens. The human body naturally hosts a variety of fungi, but when conditions are ripe, the fungus can overpopulate more healthy bacteria and cause an infection, posing a problem by making a good breeding-ground for other bacteria to invade and also by draining the body of nutrients (when present in the digestive system) by interfering with nutrient absorption.

Conditions that can lead to fungal infections include but are not limited to:

- Lack of hygiene

- Excessive hygiene (washing with soap *too* frequently)

- Consuming prescription antibiotics
- Over-use of herbal essential oils
- Over-consumption of sugar or the presence of diabetes
- AIDS/HIV
- Consumption or topical use of steroids
- Overheating
- Wet environment
- Inhalation of fungal spores

Once, when I was working on a farm, I broke open a bale of hay to throw it onto a tractor. To my surprise, the inside of the bale was completely moldy and a cloud of grayish-blue mold burst into the air. It caused a nasty infection in my lungs; I came down with a fever and for weeks suffered severe laryngitis. Mold on foods, books, and especially in damp houses are primary causes of illness, and fungi can infect the soft tissues (eyes, sinuses, throat, vagina, gastrointestinal tract) and any exposed areas such as the skin with invasive hair and nail diseases. Long-term damage from mold infections can be serious and can require hospitalization. Most fungal infections start in the lungs or on the skin, also in the vagina and the mouth. Common fungal infections include athlete's foot, ringworm, and *Candida albicans* (or yeast), called thrush in a baby's mouth. In addition to herbs previously mentioned, including garlic, cayenne, calendula, clove, tea tree, rosemary, sage, cinnamon, eucalyptus, and oregano, consider:

- **pau d'arco** (*Tabebuia impetiginosa*): laboratory studies indicate the chemicals, particularly the anthraquinones, have a "moderate" and "strong" action against *Helicobacter pylori*.[55] The inner

---

55   Park, Hyun-Kyung, and Sung-Eun (2006).

bark of the pau d'arco tree is used traditionally as an anti-inflammatory and antipathogenic for bacterial and fungal infections.

- **yarrow** (*Achillea millefolium*): antibacterial, antifungal, and astringent, yarrow is a warming diaphoretic and can be used effectively in cases of fungal infection leading to fever.

## Fungi and Antifungal Formulas

### A FORMULA FOR A SKIN FUNGAL INFECTION (AS A TEA TO DRINK)

› 2 parts echinacea

› 1 part sage

› 1 part pau d'arco

› 1 part prickly ash

### A FORMULA FOR A SKIN FUNGAL INFECTION (AS A SALVE, LINIMENT, OR RINSE)

› 2 parts pau d'arco

› 1 part sage

› 1 part calendula

› 1 part yarrow

### A FORMULA FOR A VAGINAL YEAST INFECTION (*CANDIDA ALBICANS*) (AS A TEA TO DRINK)

› 2 parts nettle

› 1 part pau d'arco

› 1 part calendula

› 1 part raspberry leaf

### A FORMULA FOR A VAGINAL YEAST INFECTION (AS A DOUCHE)

› 2 parts calendula

› 1 part pau d'arco

> › 1 part raspberry leaf

> › 1 part yarrow

## Parasites and Antiparasitic Herbs

Antiparasitic herbs kill parasites, including pinworms, tapeworm, lice, mites, and even malaria and giardia. Parasites are common pests that invade a host and live off it, using the host's flesh as food or a breeding ground, or both. Parasites can cause severe symptoms including digestive upset, gas, bloating, rashes, fever, diarrhea, vomiting, itching—or they can exist in the human body without causing any symptoms at all.

Scientists have long understood the defense that certain white cells produce against parasites, but around 2008 it became increasingly clear that a particular white blood cell, the eosinophil, actually has a profound defense position against parasites. This cell, which represents only 1 percent of all white blood cells, can identify an "invading" or foreign cell and will then "hurl" nearby mitochondrial DNA particles as well as toxic proteins (that they store within their cellular lining) at the bacteria, effectively entangling the bacteria in a net.[56] Since most eosinophils live at the borders of the gut, their action is helpful in keeping parasitic infections at bay. However, it appears that many allergic reactions, including asthma, may be worsened by the actions of the eosinophil, whose hurling techniques of toxic proteins may damage soft tissues in the proximity (such as in the lungs), thereby triggering allergic responses. Does this mean asthma may in fact be precipitated by parasitic infections? It's possible and worth considering in cases of chronic lung infections or asthma. The herbalist would want to consider adding bronchial support herbs as tier 3 in the formula, such as pleurisy root, mullein, or elderflower.

---

56   Nizet and Rothenberg (2008).

Other parasitic infections are bacterial. Giardia is a bacterial parasitic infection of the gut, often experienced when drinking fouled or contaminated water. It causes intense pain and spasms in the gut, and produces fever, vomiting, and extreme diarrhea as the body tries to eliminate the offending organism. The person needs digestive support, emotional support, direct parasite-removal, and immune support, in addition to extra liquids lost through emesis.

Common antiparasitic herbs include:

- **wormwood** (*Artemisia absinthium*) and **mugwort** (*Artemisia vulgare*): these herbs belong to the lovely and silvery *Artemisia* genus, and are renowned for their extremely bitter taste. In fact, most vermifuge (antiparasitic) herbs are very bitter and are best taken as tinctures.

- **walnut hull** (*Juglans nigra*): the green outer hull surrounding the edible walnut is harvested, turning the hands dark green in the process. Long used in European, North American, and South American herbal medicine for treating an array of fungal infections, both topically and digestive, walnut hull tastes bitter.

- **rue** (*Ruta graveolens*): included in bitter cordials, rue rids the body of parasitic worms and bacteria, both topically and in the digestive tract. Use with caution topically as both the fresh and dried plant material can cause an allergic rash in susceptible people.

- **garlic** (*Allium sativum*) and **cayenne** (*Capsicum* spp.): strong antimicrobials; great care should be exercised in their use. I avoid using these herbs with very young children (age four or younger), and use caution when suggesting these herbs internally. Garlic, of course, is a food, and its addition to the diet is welcome in raw form (it loses its bactericidal potency as well as its cholesterol-lowering properties when cooked).

*Parasites and Antiparasitic Formulas*

### A Formula for Giardia (as a tea or tincture)

> 2 parts sage

> 1 part garlic

> 1 part cramp bark

> 1 part chamomile

### Another Formula for Giardia (as a tea or tincture)

> 2 parts lemon balm

> 1 part goldenseal

> 1 part sage

> 1 part slippery elm

> ½ part fennel

### A Formula for Head Lice
### (as a topical wash or wrap to be covered with cellophane)

> 2 parts calendula

> 1 part tea tree

> 1 part rosemary

> 1 part sage

### A Formula for External Parasites (as a witch hazel topical rinse)

> 2 parts tea tree oil

> 1 part peppermint oil

> 1 part eucalyptus oil

> 1 part oregano oil

> Combine 10–20 drops of oil with ½ cup witch hazel extract (from the pharmacy). Cover the hair, making sure to avoid the eyes. Cover with a cap or towel and leave on several hours, or as long as possible. Rinse well.

### Viruses and Antiviral Herbs

Compared to viruses, bacteria seem tame. We can kill bacteria with herbal, over-the-counter, and prescription medication. But we can hardly touch viruses. To begin with, they are extremely small—about one one-hundredth the size of the average bacterium. Secondly, their uncanny ability to sabotage a cell and then replicate their RNA and DNA inside the cell is quick, efficient, and deadly: the proteins on the outside of a virus match up with those on a human cell, "unlock" it, invade it, and hide inside safe from detection from the human's immune system. While hidden, the virus replicates its own RNA and DNA, effectively overtaking and hijacking the cell's organelles. The virus duplicates itself so frequently and swiftly that the human cell soon has no choice but to burst—spewing its contents of new, fresh viruses into the human tissue or bloodstream where new sabotage quickly takes place. Because of its ability to hide within our own cells while replicating, the virus can appear to lie "dormant," revealing itself as an illness at a later stage. This is known as "viral eclipse" and seems to be common in such viral and post-viral illnesses such as Epstein-Barr (a herpes virus that causes mononucleosis), chicken pox (with its accompanying shingles), chronic fatigue immune deficiency syndrome, and herpes virus number 6 (HSV6). Other viral infections include colds, influenza, measles, mumps, rubella, croup, cytomegalovirus, meningitis, West Nile Virus, hepatitis, cold sores or herpes, encephalitis, polio, rabies, HIV and AIDS, and dengue fever, and we are even now beginning to understand some forms of gastric and peptic ulcers originally thought to be caused by stress.

Immune modulators stimulate the body's T-suppressor cells, and immuno-adjuvants increase the body's production of antibodies, leading to a presumably stronger immune response to perceived (and recognized) invaders. [57]

Antiviral herbs interrupt or destroy the virus's ability to sabotage a healthy cell and replicate itself. With the exception of echinacea and a few others, the study of antiviral herbs (in the greater context of antimicrobial herbs) is lagging and much needs to be understood about exactly how these plants work. Holistically, it is important to treat viral infection with all the body systems in mind, not just the lymphocytes or killer T cells. For instance, because it is crucial for the body's immune system to recognize, destroy, and remove foreign cells from the body, the elimination systems must be fully functional. Supporting the liver, kidneys, and digestive tract during a viral infection is just as important as supplying antiviral herbs, otherwise secondary infections can present themselves in places such as the mouth, throat, and skin. Additionally, recognizing the ill-effects of immunodeficiency and getting proper allopathic treatment can be invaluable; repeated infections, longer duration, pain, and spreading infections warrant evaluation and skilled diagnosis.

Common antiviral herbs include:

- **echinacea** (*Echinacea angustifolia*): some echinacea compounds inhibit an enzyme used by many viruses to break down cell walls in plants (and presumably our cell membranes); echinacea contains volatile oils, amides, and polypeptides that fight staphylococcal infections, act as insecticides, and attack bacteria; these chemicals are proven to be antiviral when the person is exposed to sunlight. Many herbalists prefer to use a large dose at the first sign of illness (1 ounce of tincture in the first hour) rather than using it as a preventive.

---

57   Hoffmann (1996).

- **cinnamon, rosemary, eucalyptus:** the essential oils are inhaled in steams or prepared in a salve to be rubbed on the chest.

- **lemon balm** (*Melissa officinalis*): antiviral against the herpes simplex virus topically; useful as tea, capsule, or tincture for fever and influenza.

- **licorice** (*Glycyrrhiza glabra*): the glycerrhetinic acid in licorice root is used in the treatment of peptic ulcers. It is also an excellent anti-inflammatory, antioxidant, and antibacterial. It is used as an antiviral against EBV, HIV, herpes, SARS, and influenza. [58]

- **ginseng** (*Panax ginseng*): suppresses the inflammation phase of influenza.

- **juniper berries** (*Juniperus* spp.): high in volatile oils, these seed cones are traditionally included in European and North American cold and flu preparations (avoid in kidney disease and pregnancy).

- **skullcap** (*Scutellaria baicalensis*): Chinese skullcap is anxiolytic and used to treat HIV, leukemia, hepatitis, and influenza.

Herbalists should also consider using bitter melon and quercetin-containing foods, fruits and herbs. Quercetin is a flavonoid that helps the body fight infection.

Chemically, those herbs containing glycoproteins (oligosaccharide lectins) and polysaccharides seem to be the most effective at combating viral infections. Poke root (*Phytolacca* spp.) contains lectins, though use caution when using poke because it can produce hallucinations and stomach upset when used internally. Originally studied from a food perspective and grouped with sugars and carbohydrates, certain polysaccharides are

---

58   Clare (2012).

now being recognized as being able to activate lymphocyte (white blood cell) production, increase serum proteins and interferon production, and even stimulate phagocytosis, which is the process by which white blood cells "eat" or consume the invading bacteria, rendering it harmless. Immune enhancing polysaccharide herbs include Siberian ginseng, licorice, saw palmetto, the seaweed bladderwrack, and astragalus.

Allopathic medicine has had the most success with antiviral drugs called nucleoside analogues that deceive viruses into using fake DNA to replicate within a cell; the fake DNA is missing key parts called hydroxyl groups, effectively ending the virus's attempt at DNA/RNA replication and leading to its death. To my knowledge, we do not yet know of any herbs that perform this particular function; antiviral herbal medicine relies instead on using saccharide-rich plant extracts to boost white blood cell performance.

## *Viruses and Antiviral Formulas*
### A FORMULA FOR INFLUENZA

- › 2 parts lemon balm
- › 1 part garlic
- › 1 part rose hips
- › 1 part elderberry

### A FORMULA FOR COLD SORES (HERPES SIMPLEX)

- › 2 parts lemon balm
- › 1 part licorice
- › 1 part red clover
- › 1 part echinacea

### A Formula for Colds with Sinus Congestion (as a tincture)

› 2 parts echinacea

› 1 part horseradish root

› 1 part elderberry

› 1 part elderflower

### Another Formula for Colds with Sinus Congestion

› 2 parts elderberry

› 1 part freeze-dried nettle root

› 1 part Oregon grape root

› 1 part feverfew

### A Formula for Colds with Coughs/Chest Congestion

› 2 parts elderberry

› 1 part licorice

› 1 part sage

› 1 part mullein

## Immune Strengthening Protocols

Herbalists are often asked for a particular herb to treat an illness, and while that is not an ideal way to approach herbal healing, there are indeed herbs that directly support the human immune response and can be part of a plan to prevent and fight disease. Immune function appears to be highly influenced by exercise, especially vigorous walking in the outdoors. There is much reason to believe that exercise also stimulates the immune system to better protect against invading pathogens as well. Step one in any health or recovery regimen should be to move the body and develop a robust and enjoyable exercise plan.

Immune function may or may not be influenced by mental attitude; cultivating a positive attitude may ward off diseases by keeping the heart "light," keeping blood circulation healthy, and by the person's natural tendency to move and be active. However, plenty of "positive" people get sick, so more research should be done on the mind's perception of illness and its potential ability to remedy such illness simply by a state of being. Therefore, step two is to develop and nurture a positive sense of self-worth and well-being, especially developing habits of gratitude, joy, and feelings of success (and yes, these are *habits*).

Many herbs support our immune function and have been used historically throughout Europe, Asia, Indonesia, North America, and South America to protect against illness and strengthen the immune system. These are the long-term herbs to be used as tier 1 tonics, and they are safe to use all winter for immune support and sustenance. Most of these herbs are, not surprisingly, foods, and they are consumed in the general diet of cultures such as India, where antibacterial and immune-strengthening foods are common. In addition to astragalus, rose hips, and lemon balm, consider:

- **elderberry** (*Sambucus nigra* or *S. Canadensis*): contains triterpenes, flavonoids, and tannins. Both the berry and flower are useful for catarrhal inflammation but are also traditionally used for long-term immune support, especially for chronic asthma, bronchitis, and lung congestion.

- **spilanthes** (*Acmella oleracea*): this tinctured herb creates a tingling on the tongue, and it's considered a mild immune-function stimulant.

- **mullein** (*Verbascum thapsus*): mullein can bring great relief in times of bronchial stress. Use this as a specific for bronchial catarrh and spasms as well as a tier 1 tonic for long-term support.

- **peppermint** (*Mentha × piperita*): I often use peppermint instead of spearmint in immune formulas. I find spearmint is excellent in formulas for digestion, inflammation, and for children's remedies, but I turn to peppermint, which is stronger and more intense, for immunity. It is a strong circulatory stimulant and diaphoretic.

- **ginger** (*Zingiber officinalis*): a stimulant, but in small doses can be helpful for depression, poor circulation, and anxiety that leads to stagnation. Use short-term as a tier 3 for up to 3 weeks.

- **mushrooms:** esteemed mycologist Paul Stamets teaches there are certain fungi that have been shown in clinical in-vitro trials to powerfully boost the body's immune function and inhibit herpes simplex I and II viruses, varicella zoster virus, influenza A virus, as well as mushrooms that inhibit the replication of the human immunodeficiency virus. [59] Consider maitake (*Grifola frondosa*), shiitake (*Lentinula edodes*), and agaricus (*Agaricus blazei*) for immune-enhancing and antitumor effects.

### Immune Strengthening Formulas
#### A FORMULA FOR A COLD

> › 2 parts lemon balm

> › 1 part cayenne

> › 1 part [corollary treatment: wild cherry for cough, goldenseal for congestion, etc.]

> › 1 part sage

---

59   Stamets (2015).

## A FORMULA FOR INFLUENZA WITH FEVER

› 2 parts elderberry

› 1 part garlic

› 1 part yarrow

› 1 part prickly ash

## The Lymph System

The lymph system baffled scientists when it was discovered in the late seventeenth century. The complex lymph system (actually a part of the circulatory system) traverses our entire body, both in the internal depths and on the more superficial layers, transporting clear fluids and acting as a backup for the bacteria-fighting duties of the immune system. Lymph tissues and lymphoid follicles are associated with the immune and digestive systems and can be found in the spleen, tonsils, thymus, bone marrow, and other organs. Interestingly, lymph fluid travels in the lymphatic vessels in a one-way direction toward the heart, much as blood travels in a one-way direction from the heart, around the left side of the body, up the right side, and back to the heart. This amazing lymphatic network surrounds our cells with a sort of cleaning fluid that removes cellular and metabolic wastes for disposal, and it has the remarkable ability to trap cancerous cells and destroy them. Sometimes, though, cells are not destroyed completely and the cancer can betray the lymph system by using it to travel through the network to other nodes that can harbor secondary tumors. This can result in Hodgkin's lymphoma and non-Hodgkin's lymphoma, cancers of the lymph system.

While cancer of the lymph system is very serious and requires allopathic medical attention, herbalism has a lot to offer in the way of lymph system nourishment, immune support, and corollary support for secondary symptoms. Certain herbs nourish the lymph system to keep lymph fluids flowing freely. Herbs such as cleavers (lady's bedstraw, or *Gallium aparine*) have historically been prized for "decongesting" the lymph system and allowing the fluids to travel. (Cleavers are also used for other "drainage" issues including bladder infection, dysuria, and kidney stones.) Other herbs such as echinacea, astragalus and barberry assist the lymph system in its job of trapping and killing cancerous cells. Some studies also show that a properly functioning lymph system can also play a key role in helping overweight women regain their proper weight and in relieving pain throughout the body.

The lymph system responds well to tart fruits and vegetables, so eating cranberries and fruits or herbs high in flavonoids, malic acids, and citric acids (such as wood sorrel, spinach, apples, tamarinds) can be helpful. Other "immune-support" herbs such as astragalus, goldenseal, and poke root have been identified as powerful lymph system supporters, though caution must be used with poke as it can induce hallucinations. Astragalus, however, can be used frequently, even as a food (especially in stews and soups).

### *Lymph System Formulas*
#### A FORMULA FOR LYMPH SUPPORT (AS A TEA, TINCTURE, OR CAPSULE)
> › 2 parts astragalus
> › 2 parts cleavers
> › 1 part cranberry

## Lyme Infection

Lyme is such a quirky, prevalent, and misdiagnosed illness that I'll list it separately here with immune functions. Lyme is a tough one: it's altogether not what we think it is, despite all the tests and clinical studies. I wouldn't be surprised if, in the next twenty-five to fifty years, we realize that many of today's illnesses are actually a result of suffering from Lyme.

What is Lyme? Based on today's understanding, we believe it is caused by infection by the tiny *Borrelia bergdorferi sensu lato*, a spirochete bacterium that can live inside deer ticks and be transmitted to humans after a tick bite. Once the tick bites flesh, the *Borrelia* propels itself from the gut of the tick into the flesh and the bloodstream. The bacterium quickly multiplies and can invade joint tissues and even nervous tissues. Within ten to fifteen days of a bite, symptoms of Lyme disease can include fever, headache, stiff or sore muscles, and often a large (five inch by five inch) "bull's-eye" rash. My son was bitten at age five, and he displayed not one bulls-eye, but approximately twenty-five half-dollar sized red bull's-eyes, along with fever. Early dosing with doxycycline is recommended, as Lyme that goes untreated can cause serious and lasting impairments in the joints, the eyes, and other body systems. In addition to Lyme, other tick-borne illnesses (coinfections) with similar symptoms and prognoses include tularemia, ehrlichiosis, Rocky Mountain spotted fever, babesiosis, and the newly discovered Powassan virus.

Herbalist Stephen Buhner, arguably one of the leading experts on herbal treatment of Lyme and its coinfections, shares that Lyme may be transmitted through human fluids, such as semen and breast milk. He believes *Borrelia* has the evolutionary ability to sample human tissues and fluids to determine where its best location for infection will be.[60] Specific tier 2 herbs for Lyme include:

- **andrographis** (*Andrographis paniculata*): appears to be antispirochete and apparently crosses the blood-brain barrier. Anti-inflammatory and immune stimulant. Buhner calls it "perhaps the best primary herb to use in the treatment of Lyme disease."[61]

---

60   Buhner (2005).

61   Ibid. 78.

Can cause skin rashes and side effects, though it is a natural liver-support and waste remover for Lyme and other infections.

- **stephania** (*Stephania* spp.): with a wide variety of species—each acting slightly differently—stephania is worth considering especially for nerve inflammation. Useful for ocular borreliosis and Lyme infection disparaging neural connections.

- **Japanese knotweed** (*Polygonum cuspidatum*): contains the chemical resveratrol that halts the inflammatory response. Modulates immune response and is a key herb against Lyme and all its coinfections. Especially important for brain and nerve inflammation in Lyme. [62]

- **cat's claw** (*Uncaria guianensis, U. tomentosa*): a tropical vine found throughout South America and Asia, cat's claw has been used by South American Indian cultures for centuries and is now undergoing trials to gauge its efficacy as an anti-inflammatory. Scientists believe cat's claw may suppress tumor necrosis factor (TNF), making it a possible remedy for tumors and cancers. This anti-TNF activity is anti-inflammatory in the bowels, as well, making cat's claw a potential remedy for Crohn's disease. [63] Lyme sufferers use cat's claw to reduce the painful arthritic symptoms that accompany Lyme and its coinfections.

- **astragalus** (*Astragalus membranaceus*): high in triterpene glycosides, astragalus is noted through clinical and laboratory research as an immunostimulant, antiviral, and hepatoprotective herb. It has been shown effective against viral myocarditis and viral hepatitis and is active against tumor cells. [64]

---

62   Gilday (2013).

63   Phaneuf, Holly (2005).

64   Thompson Healthcare Inc. (2007) 57.

- **spilanthes** (*Spilanthes acmella* or *Acmella oleracea*): though tests are ongoing, spilanthes is an immune-support herb and is an antiparasitic. Known as jambu in Brazil, spilanthes is a traditional oral-infection remedy for mouth ulcers and as a flavoring agent. Herbalist Jill Stansbury mentions it may have antispirochetal effects[65], making it possibly effective for syphilis and Lyme since both diseases result from the infection of a spirochete, a corkscrew-shaped bacteria that is notorious for its ability to lay dormant in the body for long periods of time.

Corollary support tier 3 herbs include:

- **eleuthero** (*Eleutherococcus senticosus*): also called Siberian ginseng, this adaptogen supports nerve function, increases energy (without caffeine), provides long-term sustained energy, and is a pivotal tier 1 tonic or tier 3 corollary herb.
- **boneset** (*Eupatorium perfoliatum*): for deep and chronic muscle aches.
- **wild sarsaparilla** (*Aralia nudicaulis*): for fatigue.

## Lyme Infection Formulas

Each of the following formulas should be taken as capsules or powders (not teas or tinctures) with freshly dried, highly potent, organic herbs.

### A FORMULA FOR LYME WITH MUSCLE AND/OR BONE PAIN

> › 2 parts Japanese knotweed
>
> › 1 part pau d'arco
>
> › 1 part cat's claw
>
> › 1 part teasel
>
> › 1 part boneset

---

65  Stansberry and Willard (2002).

### A Formula for Lyme with immune support

> › 2 parts astragalus
> › 1 part andrographis
> › 1 part elderberry
> › 1 part eleuthero

### A Formula for Men: Lyme with fatigue and mental fog

> › 2 parts lemon balm or ginkgo
> › 1 part cat's claw
> › 1 part eleuthero
> › 1 part wild sarsaparilla

### A Formula for Women: Lyme with fatigue and mental fog

> › 2 parts lemon balm or ginkgo
> › 2 parts eleuthero
> › 1 part cat's claw
> › 1 part motherwort or ginger

Nourishing and supporting the immune system can be accomplished using the antimicrobial herbs outlined here, making sure common sense, proper diet, and a proactive lifestyle are a priority. Improving and supporting immune function is a life-enhancing practice. Be open to new herbs, or in new combinations, as each person you work with is different, has unique needs, and responds to herbal medicines differently.

# CHAPTER NINE

# Inflammation and Pain

Inflammation can happen anywhere in the body—the digestive system, the brain, the skin, and in the connective tissues and joints. Many of my clients want to address arthritic and rheumatic complaints in addition to other issues (or sometimes as the main issue) and often a topical application is part of the solution.

Inflammation is the body's natural response to a variety of triggers, such as toxins in the food, a physical wound or injury, or in less frequent cases, an apparently allergic reaction to the body's own tissues (such as in rheumatoid arthritis). In this chapter we'll address inflammation as it relates to muscles, nerves, and injuries, as well as the pain that often accompanies swelling and mobility restriction.

In a 4-tier formula, focus is given to nourishing herbs that alleviate nervous tension (nervine tonics) and to corollary herbs that support the digestive/elimination system since the body's production of proteins in response to (especially autoimmune) inflammation is a potential source of pain. Making sure the body can process and quickly eliminate these proteins is part of an overall strategy for reducing inflammation. Also, hepatics (liver-supporting herbs) are good tier 3 herbs so the body's efforts at processing spent proteins, hormones, and other biochemicals is efficient, and circulatory herbs get the blood moving through areas of the body that seem "stagnant" due to inflammation.

Anti-inflammatory herbs are the tier 2 Specifics that address the core of the problem. These vary from culture to culture, with a wide range of botanical species providing chemical constituents that reduce swelling in human tissue. Among these are:

- **devil's claw** (*Harpagophytum procumbens*): this bitter plant originated in South Africa and is used clinically as an anti-inflammatory and analgesic for arthritis.

- **arnica** (*Arnica montana*): clinically proven to relieve pain and joint stiffness, to assist in wound healing, and to be analgesic when applied topically. [66] Most trials involve homeopathic arnica but infused oil arnica applications topically have years of effective and safe household use. Arnica should never be used in tincture form, only topically or in homeopathic form.

- **wild yam** (*Dioscorea villosa*): especially as an antispasmodic for pelvic, uterine, and gastric inflammation or cramps

- **Jamaican dogwood** (*Piscidia erythrina* or *P. piscipula*): as a sedative and spasmolytic for insomnia due to pain, and for anxiety that causes muscle constriction. Beware of side effects that may include nausea and dizziness; this is a strong herb to be used with caution and good sense

---

66  Thompson Healthcare Inc. (2007), 45–47.

- **willow** (*Salix* spp.) and **meadowsweet** (*Filipendula* spp.): with their high salicin content, these are anodynes for rheumatism and pain, and especially for diseases accompanied by fever, headaches and inflammatory pain. Note: never give salicin-containing herbs to children younger than seventeen who present with fever because of the danger of Reye's syndrome.

- **lobelia** (*Lobelia inflata*): also called pukeweed or Indian tobacco, lobelia is a strong antispasmodic for muscles, lungs, and uterine cramps. Determining correct dosage is key as the herb can produce nausea or vomiting.

- **turmeric** (*Curcuma longa*): taken internally, the spice or condiment normally used in Asian cuisine is a well-known anti-inflammatory for muscle and joint pain.

- **valerian** (*Valeriana officinalis*): a sedative and anxiolytic useful for stress that causes muscle constriction, as well as for inflammation of the uterus, neuralgia, colic, and headache. Generally considered sleep-inducing and even soporific.

- **cramp bark** (*Viburnum opulus*): a useful antispasmodic especially for uterine cramps.

## Topical Applications

Also, certain herbs can be used topically as especially warming and soothing external remedies. Formulations called compresses (fomentations), poultices, salves, liniments, and ointments use the following herbs to best effect, making sure they are used exclusively externally and in a dilution of water, witch hazel, or oil. These include:

- **ginger** (*Zingiber officinale*)
- **mustard** (*Brassica* spp.)
- **arnica** (*Arnica montana*)

- **yarrow** (*Achillea millefolium*)

- **plantain** (*Plantago major* or *P. lanceolata*)

- **violet** (*Viola* spp.)

- **wintergreen** (*Gaultheria procumbens*)

- **cinnamon** (*Cinnamomum* spp.)

- **cayenne** (*Capsicum* spp.)

As these are warming and stimulating, use caution in their application, and avoid soft delicate tissues (such as the eyes and the vagina) and open wounds.

Tier 1 tonics for rheumatic complaints include many of the nourishing herbs previously mentioned, such as the mineral-rich herb oatstraw or oats milky tops, vervain, chamomile, eleuthero, rhodiola, holy basil, and lemon balm.

### Topical Inflammation and Pain Formulas
#### A FORMULA FOR ARTHRITIS (AS A TEA, TINCTURE, OR CAPSULE)

› 2 parts oats milky tops

› 1 part devil's claw

› 1 part prickly ash bark

› 1 part cramp bark

#### A FORMULA FOR ARTHRITIS (AS A TOPICAL LINIMENT OR SALVE)

› 2 parts arnica extract

› 1 part wintergreen oil

› 1 part eucalyptus or Scots pine (*Pinus sylvestris*) oil

› 1 part dandelion leaf

## A Formula for Arthritis with Insomnia
## (as a tea, tincture, or capsule)

› 2 parts skullcap

› 1 part Jamaican dogwood

› 1 part white willow

› ½ part lavender

## Another Formula for Arthritis with Insomnia
## (as a tea, tincture, or capsule)

› 2 parts chamomile

› 2 parts valerian

› 1 part meadowsweet

› 1 part hops

## A Formula for Arthritis with Insomnia
## (as a topical liniment or salve)

› 2 parts lavender oil

› 1 part arnica extract

› 1 part mullein leaf extract

› ½ part dandelion leaf extract

## Another Formula for Arthritis with Insomnia
## (as a topical liniment or salve)

› 2 parts Scots pine

› 1 part black mustard seed

› Diluted with a carrier oil or used as a plaster

# Internal Inflammation

We've discussed topical or sub-topical inflammation such as arthritis, rheumatism, and pain in the musculoskeletal system or on the skin. Let's turn our attention to internal instances of inflammation that can cause pain or secondary illness to the body's organs.

Many illnesses cause internal inflammation: everything from indigestion to chronic Lupus will result in inflammation of an organ or organ system. Like topical inflammation, internal inflammation is often accompanied by pain, but vague internal pain can be particularly worrisome and can bring on anxiety and frustration. In addition to the herbs outlined here, consider a person's mental state of mind and use cooling or soothing herbs as needed in addition to the anti-inflammatory tier 2 Specifics. Because internal inflammation can be triggered by such a wide range of causes, we will focus on one in particular as an example of herbal formulary for such instances: chronic pelvic pain.

## Chronic Pelvic Pain

Long-term pain experienced in the uterine region can signal any number of diseases, which is why pain that lasts more than a few months and is not cyclic (linked to the menstrual cycle) must be shared with your health care provider. Chronic pelvic pain (CPP) can be indicative of pelvic inflammatory disease (PID), adhesions, fibroids, endometriosis, cystitis, dysmenorrhea, and even autoimmune diseases. Typical symptoms include constipation or diarrhea, dysmenorrhea, leg pain, lower back pain, abdominal "heaviness," and vaginal/uterine spasms. Cardiovascular issues must be considered and personal history of abuse and current relationships should be evaluated to rule out a psychogenic cause. Once a skilled diagnosis has been made, herbs may be considered for symptom reduction and nourishment filling every tier of the formula. In addition to the tier 2 Specifics already mentioned for external inflammation, such as cramp bark, consider:

- **angelica** (*Angelica sinensis*): also called dong quai, this fragrant herb is used for respiratory and digestive complaints and can be a tier 2 specific for pelvic congestion and uterine cramps.
- **corydalis** (*Corydalis cava*): as a sedative, hypnotic, and analgesic, the roots ease spasms and pain in the pelvis that preclude sleep, especially for women with CPP. Gaining popularity for use in Parkinson's disease, as its complex alkaloids show antispasmodic activity. [67]
- **black cohosh** (*Actaea racemosa*): analgesic, antispasmodic.
- **wild yam** (*Dioscorea villosa*): antispasmodic, especially for pelvic congestion.
- **motherwort** (*Leonurus cardiaca*): antispasmodic to the digestive tract, nervine, bitter. Can be used as a tier 1 tonic or a tier 3 corollary.
- **ginger** (*Zingiber officinale*): antispasmodic, vasodilator, warming aromatic. Can be used topically or internally.
- **chamomile** (*Matricaria recutita*): nervine, bitter. Excellent tier 1 tonic.
- **raspberry** (*Rubus ideaus*): nervine, tonic, astringent. Particularly helpful in cases of pelvic congestion, post-partum pain and depression, and fibroids.
- **turmeric** (*Curcuma longa*): antispasmodic, anti-inflammatory.

### Chronic Pelvic Pain Formulas
#### A FORMULA FOR CHRONIC PELVIC PAIN
> › 2 parts motherwort
> › 1 part wild yam

---

67 Thompson Healthcare Inc. (2007), 232.

> › 1 part ginger

> › 1 part red raspberry

## ANOTHER FORMULA FOR CHRONIC PELVIC PAIN

> › 2 parts chamomile

> › 1 part dong quai (*Angelica sinensis*)

> › 1 part licorice

> › 1 part valerian

The herbal repertoire abounds in herbs that relieve inflammation (anti-inflammatories) and ease pain (analgesic or anodyne). Using these as tier 2 Specifics allows us to place other herbs in other tiers, including nervous system support herbs as tier 1 tonics; digestive, carminative, and bitter herbs as tier 3 corollary; warming and circulatory tonics as tier 3 corollary; and digestive or uterine herbs as tier 4 Vehicle, where needed. Keep in mind that internal inflammation can also be eased using external remedies such as compresses.

# CHAPTER TEN

# The Skin–
# Wounds and First Aid

The skin does a lot: as the largest organ of the body, it is composed of the epidermis, the dermis, and the hypodermis. The skin performs a variety of functions: it protects us from pathogens, dirt, debris, and damage; it controls evaporation of fluids, allowing us to sweat (something dogs cannot do), which is tied to our adrenal system; it keeps water in, which is a useful thing to remember when you're addressing burn wounds and trauma victims, and it allows us to sense the outside world through touch and the perception of temperature. Because it is connected to blood vessels and muscle cells, the skin helps regulate internal body temperature;

The skin gives us signals through the day indicating our environment, who or what might be close by, and even—if we know how to interpret—information about what's going on in our internal organs, including our digestive and circulatory systems. Many healers palpate the skin as a key diagnostic tool. Touching the body to detect heat, sweat, swelling, moistness or drying is a method long used by Tibetan, Chinese, and Ayurvedic practitioners.

The skin is both easy to evaluate and difficult to master. Each person looks different, which is why a holistic approach to *both* diagnosis and treatment is essential. Taking a person's entire experience into account (physical, dietary, mental, emotional, spiritual, and future perspective) is key to learning what herbs and foods may best help complete this person's picture of health. That, after all, is what herbalists and other healing arts practitioners do—we don't prescribe, nor do we tell a person what he or she needs. We facilitate as a person learns to feel their best. Killing microorganisms is secondary. Attaining perfect health is also secondary—a philosophy that may surprise some people, especially those who look at herbal healing as an adjunct of allopathic medicine and another method through which he or she can attain the "magic bullet." There is no magic bullet here, and the primary emphasis of any herbalist's work with a client should be to help that client discover his or her optimum experience.

## Eczema, Psoriasis, Rashes, and Topical Yeast Infection

Eczema and psoriasis are difficult to evaluate and remedy simply because they affect a wide range of people (aged, elderly, babies, men, women, smokers, vegetarians) and because they appear in various places on the body, look different on each person, and can be triggered by a wide range of factors.

Each may be only superficial (the result of direct external contact with an irritant or toxin) or they may result from an inner imbalance in the liver or digestive system. The skin eruptions (inflammation, rashes, and itching) are symptoms (expressions) of a much deeper imbalance in the gastrointestinal, hepatic, nervous, or reproductive systems. The cause of eczema frequently lies in the digestive tract; clients suffering from eczema or related rashes should be examined for liver health and should explore food allergies in addition to exploring antifungal herbs.

I recognize the fear and concern of those dealing with these bizarre and abnormal irritations, especially when the eruptions occur frequently and "for no apparent reason." Some are severe and can appear in alarming places, such as the eyelids. Sometimes children scratch themselves raw, and even adults are so bothered by the itching they must put socks on their hands at night to keep from making the infection worse. There are a number of plants from which you can make effective remedies for both external and internal relief, and we'll go into these in detail shortly. Eczema and psoriasis begin inside the body but express themselves through the skin (and other organs).

What's the difference between eczema and psoriasis? In general, eczema is characterized by oozing, red, blister-like pustules that itch and often crust over. These red, yellow, or orange eczema blisters are usually found in the warm, moist areas of the body: in the creases of the elbows and knees, the folds of the neck, or in the navel, though they can also be flat and found on more dry places, such as cheeks and the backs of hands and fingers, where the blisters appear swollen, dry, and are extremely tender. Eczema is thought to have two causes: an allergy to an external irritant (such as industrial solvents, dyes, soaps, shampoos, or even heat), and diet. Many people clear eczema by removing dairy, wheat, or sugar from their diet.

Psoriasis is characterized by gray-colored, dry scales usually found on the dry, bony parts of the body—the elbows, kneecaps, or ribs. Something triggers the skin cells to proliferate more quickly than they can be shed, and these cells build up in one spot, creating an uncomfortable mass of skin and scales. Most remedies involve changing the diet, moisturizing the area, and gently scrubbing to remove the scales. Herbalists should also consider nervine tonics as stress appears to be a factor.

Yeast is normal both internally and externally; *Candida albicans*, a type of fungal yeast, lives in the gut, throughout the digestive system, in the vagina, and on the surface of the skin. Yeast becomes a problem when it overproliferates often due to antibiotic or other drug use, or due to the intake of excessively sugary and starchy foods. Externally, "good" microbes are washed away (or killed by solvents, harsh chemicals, dyes, and contaminants), or excretory systems including the liver are unable to remove excess yeast through normal means.

General protocols for eczema, psoriasis, and yeast infection include:

1. **Relax.** Stress can trigger hormone production and responses from the pituitary and adrenal glands. These responses are the body's protection from perceived attack and are meant to keep us safe, but they often go ignored and lead to chronic stress symptoms. Complementary therapies include salt baths, massage using lavender oils, daily meditations, guided stress reduction therapies, visits with friends, and breaks from work.

2. **Remove dairy, simple carbohydrates, and fermented foods.** Yeast (especially *Candida albicans*) thrives on dairy, sugars, and refined grains such as wheat.

3. **Take acidophilus,** especially *Lactobacillus acidophilus*. Probiotics protect the gastrointestinal tract by repopulating living organisms that normally inhabit the body, and they improve digestion and liver function. Find probiotics at health food stores and in unsweetened yogurt.

4. **Care for the liver.** As a detoxifying organ (along with the skin, kidneys, lungs, colon, and lymph system), the liver is tasked with removing harmful or waste substances from the body. Hepatic herbs such as milk thistle and dandelion are tier 3 corollary herbs in many formulas.

5. **Avoid harsh, chemical-laden environments.** Factory workers, laundry workers, nurses, and even artisans are constantly subjecting their bodies to contact with contaminants including bleach, paints, dyes, blood, astringents, perfumes, antibiotics, intense

soaps, and other chemicals that destroy the normal balance of bacteria on the skin, enabling yeast to flourish.

There are a number of herbal methods for addressing eczema, psoriasis, and yeast. The goal in treating eczema should be to soothe the client (both the skin and the emotions), and to bring the body's microbial environment into balance. Apply emollient herbs to the skin to soothe the itch, redness, and heat. These herbs include:

- calendula
- chickweed
- red clover
- marshmallow

All of these herbs are safe to use on the youngest infant; either make a tea from the herbs, dip a soft cloth in the tea, wring it slightly, and apply it to the affected area, or chop the herbs, infuse them in oil, and melt with beeswax to make a salve that can be smeared on the area. Also consider applying fresh unsweetened yogurt to the affected skin, as this will introduce *Lactobacillium* directly to the area where a yeast infection may be present.

Antibacterial and antifungal herbs reduce the infection; these include the mildest, such as calendula, raspberry seed, black cumin seed (*Nigella*), and kukui nut (*Aleurites moluccanus*) oil, to the strongest, which in my experience is pau d'arco:

- **pau d'arco** (*Tabebuia* spp.): the bark of this South American tree has been used by Brazilian healers and in the construction industry for planks, timber, and decking. In the construction trade, the wood is called ipe (pronounced ee-pay), and it is incredibly hard. I've attempted to reuse ipe wood we removed from a deck at our house, and I couldn't even hammer a nail into it. This denseness and hardiness first alerted people to its potential application in medicine; the wood is highly resistant to bacterial infection, disease, and decay. Today, lapacho tea is made from the shredded bark of certain *Tabebuia* species (pink ipe), while Taheebo tea is made from the bark of other species. Pau d'arco medicinal tisanes are regarded for their pleasant flavor and for their ability to address a wide range of bacterial and fungal infections internally and externally. I also believe this herb will prove invaluable in the treatment of Lyme disease. (Caution: do not use pau d'arco when pregnant; do not use this herb for infants or very young children under the age of 4; use it with caution and under the supervision of an herbalist if you are breastfeeding, and be aware of side effects, which can include vomiting.)

Tier 3 corollary herbs include those that tone and nourish the liver so that this metabolizing and excretory organ can perform at peak capacity. Hepatic (liver nourishing) herbs have a long history of safety and efficacy, both in America and Europe. Apple cider vinegar is the menstruum of choice when making tinctures with hepatic herbs. They function best when consumed as foods (in stews, soups, and chopped into salads):

- **dandelion** (*Taraxacum vulgare*): nutrient-rich, tasty, and bitter. Dandelion stimulates bile production and may help against certain cancers. It is anti-inflammatory, mildly anodyne (analgesic), and is a well-known diuretic, helpful for conditions of urinary and kidney disease. The root is high in iron, essential in the production of red blood cells.

- **milk thistle** (*Carduus* or *Silybum marianum*): clinically proven as a hepatoprotective in the treatment of viral or alcohol-induced cirrhosis. [68]

---

68   Thompson Healthcare Inc. (2007), 578.

- **yellow dock** (*Rumex crispus*): a traditional liver herb; not a long-term tonic because it contains oxalates.

- **burdock** (*Arctium lappa*): Called gobo in China, burdock is a common wildflower whose edible root can be chopped and stirred into soups and stews. Both the root and the seeds are used traditionally as alterative and hepatic remedies.

- **cleavers** (*Galium aparine*) for its beneficial effect on the lymph system, another excretory and highly immune supportive system of the body closely attuned to the function of the liver.

### *Eczema, Psoriasis, Rashes, and Topical Yeast Infection Formulas*
#### A FORMULA FOR ECZEMA (AS A TINCTURE OR TEA TO DRINK)
> - 2 parts dandelion leaf and root
> - 1 part pau d'arco inner bark
> - 1 part calendula blossom

#### ANOTHER FORMULA FOR ECZEMA (AS A TINCTURE OR TEA TO DRINK)
> - 2 parts dandelion leaf and root
> - 1 part black cumin seed
> - 1 part calendula
> - ½ part ginger

#### ANOTHER FORMULA FOR ECZEMA (AS A RINSE, SALVE, LINIMENT, OR OIL)
> - 2 parts pau d'arco inner bark
> - 1 part chickweed
> - 1 part black cumin seed

### Another Formula for Eczema (as a rinse, salve, liniment, or oil)

› 2 parts calendula

› 1 part plantain

› 1 part raspberry seed oil

› 1 part marshmallow root

### Another Formula for Psoriasis (as a tincture or tea to drink)

› 2 parts nettle

› 1 part lemon balm

› 1 part rose petal

› 1 part chickweed

### Another Formula for Psoriasis (as an oil or salve)

› 2 parts marshmallow root

› 1 part plantain

› 1 part red clover

› 1 part calendula

## First Aid: Healing Burns

Burns can range in severity from a mild sunburn to a fourth degree burn, in which the burn compromises or destroys not only the epidermal or underlying tissues but also extends deeper to affect muscle tissues and/or bones. Every degree of burn in between is dangerous and should be assessed by qualified health care practitioners, especially since burns can change over time, when what is initially thought to be a mild superficial burn turns into a deeper (and riskier) injury. Along with burns come the corollary issues of infection, and possibly shock, cardiovascular problems, and with very serious burns, the possibility of death. Always treat burns with great respect and seek immediate attention, especially if there is any display by the burn victim of shock, confusion, hyperventilation, excessive blood loss, etc.

This book will address mild burns that can be attended to at home, using common sense and the skills necessary to properly clean and bandage a wound. The herbalist's job in addressing burn injuries is to:

- Treat the person as a person, and not as an injury;
- Address the person's mental health with assurance, calm, peaceful attention—all the while maintaining a realistic picture of the injury both to the patient and to any medical personnel;
- Maintain strict cleanliness;
- Provide emollient and/or sanitizing herbal applications to the wound;
- Provide nervine tonic herbs for the patient to address emotions;
- Provide analgesic herbs for the patient to address pain;
- Provide drinking water and electrolytes, as needed;
- Assist the patient with bandaging and mobility.

Our herbal heritage offers a wide range of healing herbs for burn-damaged tissues. A number of herbs create a mucilaginous "gel" when steeped in water, and this oozy gel can be applied directly to mild burn wounds. Specifically, marshmallow (*Malva sylvestris*) and plantain (*Plantago major*) are useful. Chop the mallow root or the plantain leaf coarsely, and simmer it lightly in a shallow pan of water. The longer it simmers, the more gelatinous the water will become; after 20 or 30 minutes, the pan will contain a slimy liquid. Carefully skim out the herbal matter and use this slimy liquid as the healing medium on the burn, either placing the skin in direct contact with the (cooled) pan of water, or soaking a soft cloth in the pan, gently wringing it, and placing this directly on the burn. (Flannel is best, cotton is good, wool is too coarse—be careful of any hairs.)

Also consider lavender (*Lavandula angustifolia*) blossoms and leaves, as lavender is a soothing and calming herb with essential oils that have been shown to reduce the formation of scar tissue. But be careful about using it on fresh burns as it may be too intense, and never use essential oils directly on freshly burned tissue.

Be aware of other potential issues such as headache, vomiting, accelerated heartbeat, loss of electrolytes, and shock. Shock should be addressed by a qualified health care practitioner (at the emergency room), but these other issues may be carefully supervised at home. Headache responds well to analgesic herbs such as willow (*Salix* spp.), meadowsweet (*Filipendula ulmaria*), lavender (*Lavandula angustifolia*), and feverfew (*Tanacetum parthenium* or *Chrysanthemum parthenium*). Other soothing remedies can include a cup of warm chamomile tea (*Matricaria recutita*) to soothe the nerves and calm the stomach if the person is likely to "freak out" or vomit. Topically, as the burn heals and the skin reforms (depending on the severity of the burn, this could take several days), other soothing herbs can be applied topically, including calendula, chickweed, comfrey, red clover, lavender, lemon balm, elder leaf, elderflower, and even yarrow (once the wound is dry and all blisters have disappeared). The best applications for these herbs are in soothing oils (including olive, safflower, sunflower, wheat germ, hemp, or sweet almond oils), or in honey.

It's easy to prepare a medicinal honey for topical application. Honey has been used for centuries in many countries as an immediate first-aid remedy for burns, since it is a humectant (it retains moisture), and it creates a natural barrier on the skin, protecting the work of regenerating skin tissue underneath. Honey can be contaminated by yeasts or salmonella bacteria, but in clean environments the external application of fresh clean honey is generally safe. To infuse the honey, crush or chop the herbs (use those listed above), place them in a clean, dry saucepan, and submerge them in honey. Allow to sit, covered, overnight, or for several hours. Gently bring to a simmer—only enough to reliquefy the honey—and strain out the herbs. Bottle the honey into a sterilized jar (canning jars work well for this), and apply the honey to the burn. Such infused honey is delicious and can also be eaten, and because of its immune-stimulating properties may be a wonderful addition to the diet of the burn victim during recuperation.

### *Burn Formulas*

#### A FORMULA FOR MILD BURNS (AS A TINCTURE OR TEA TO DRINK)

› 2 parts skullcap

› 1 part red clover

› 1 part oatstraw

#### A FORMULA FOR MILD BURNS
#### (AS A SALVE, OIL, COMPRESS, OR INFUSED HONEY)

› 2 parts marshmallow

› 1 part aloe vera

› 1 part red clover

#### ANOTHER FORMULA FOR MILD BURNS
#### (AS A SALVE, OIL, COMPRESS OR INFUSED HONEY)

› 2 parts red clover

› 1 part plantain

› 1 part fresh lavender

## First Aid: Healing Wounds

Wounds require a slightly different healing tactic than burns. Wounds include scrapes, cuts, bruises, lacerations, punctures, splinters, gouges, and "strawberries," all of which can call for various actions from the *materia medica*. Punctures are especially risky since they can push anaerobic bacteria deep into the tissues, leading to tetanus infection. Deep puncture wounds require medical evaluation and cleaning using an iodine antiseptic or hydrogen peroxide and a wash of antibacterial herbs such as goldenseal, oregano, or thyme.

Most wounds can be addressed using the following actions:

## Vulneraries

Most wounds involve bleeding and the compression or tearing of tissues, which aggravates the muscles underneath, tears nerve endings, and exposes tender tissue to air. Vulneraries "sew" skin tissues back together (comfrey and yarrow) or kill germs (goldenseal or thyme). Every culture has its favorite wound herbs: British-Israeli Gypsy herbalist and veterinarian Juliette de Bairacli Levy loved using rosemary[69]; yarrow is a favorite in Western herbal medicine because it is healing to torn tissues and styptic, stopping blood flow quickly. Etymologically, if you are vulnerable, you can be hurt, so a wound healing herb is called a *vulnerary*.

## Astringent

These herbs dry up a wet, oozing, bloody, or pus-filled wound so that it can heal. Many astringents contain tannins that bind tissues together, assisting with clot formations and creating quick coverings over a wound so that contaminants cannot enter. Consider cranesbill, shepherd's purse, cinquefoil, witch hazel, goldenrod, and yarrow. It's easy to make a water-based rinse or wash with oak leaves or witch hazel leaves, once all foreign debris has been cleaned from a wound.

## Anti-inflammatory

Inflammation is the body's natural response to injury; blood rushes to the area causing swelling and heat. Where inflammation is extreme, causing pain, or interfering with other healing efforts, anti-inflammatories are

---

69   Levy (1966).

useful. Generally, cooling and calming anti-inflammatories are called for. Anti-inflammatories for burns and wounds include calendula, plantain, red clover, and violet leaf. These can be applied as a compress, a liniment, or infused in oil and used as a tier 2 specific, a tier 3 corollary, or a tier 4 Vehicle. Strong anti-inflammatories include:

- **chickweed** (*Stellaria media*): a cooling herb ideal for red, hot, and inflamed tissues. A favorite antipruritic (anti-itch) remedy, chickweed is soothing for poison ivy and itchy scabs and sores.

- **St. John's wort** (*Hypericum perforatum*): excellent for topical application as well as a tincture for nerve pain and stress.

- **comfrey leaf** (*Symphytum officinale*): a mild anti-inflammatory that "knits" together skin tissues at the wound site; do not use on deep cuts or exposed tissue.

- **arnica** (*Arnica montana*): a strong anti-inflammatory and analgesic; useful for both muscle and joint pain, bruising, and for arthritic and rheumatic conditions. Because arnica is difficult to cultivate and over-harvested in its natural habitat, use it sparingly.

## Emollient

Soothing herbs used externally to soften the skin, bring elasticity back to the skin, and cool or soothe heat and pain. Consider the anti-inflammatories mentioned above as well as aloe vera, mallow, slippery elm, lavender, red clover, elderflower, rose, and comfrey, which can only be applied once deeper serrations have been healed, since it works so quickly.

## Antibacterial

These can often be too strong for use on burns but are indicated on general wounds. Strong germ-killing herbs include goldenseal, thyme, oregano, sage, yarrow, mint, and calendula, all of which can be used in compress or liniment form (avoid making poultices for open wounds as pieces of the herb can irritate healing tissues).

### *Nervine Tonic*

As with any first aid or trauma treatment, assisting the patient with emotional stress is a large part of the holistic philosophy. It's not enough to simply disinfect the wound; it's important to ease the person back into a state of comfort and even joy after they've been through a stressful period of fear, panic, guilt, confusion, or pain, and while they're going through what can be a humiliating, stressful, or possibly even embarrassing period of recovery. Emotional stress can be alleviated with herbs in tier 1:

- **motherwort** (*Leonurus cardiaca*): this bitter can stimulate sluggish digestion and help overcome anxiety, fear, and panic.

- **lemon balm** (*Melissa officinalis*): along with ginkgo and gotu kola, lemon balm speeds blood flow to the brain, normalizes mental processes, and quickens mental clarity.

- **oatstraw** (*Avena sativa*): this long-term nerve tonic strengthens the nervous system.

- **lemon verbena** (*Aloysia citrodora*): antioxidant, soothing, fragrant and tasty as a tea in post-traumatic situations

- **skullcap** (*Scutellaria lateriflora*): mildly sedative, useful in nervous exhaustion

- **chamomile** (*Matricaria recutita*): sedative and bitter for stomach upset and nausea due to trauma

- **valerian** (*Valeriana officinalis*): sedative, eases fear and panic; can cause stomach upset; combine with hops for insomnia due to injury

- **catnip** (*Nepeta cataria*): soothing, calming, carminative. I find it especially useful for children post-trauma.

- **hops** (*Humulus lupulus*): sedative and bitter, can be taken as a tincture for panic, fear, and insomnia following an injury

- **passionflower** (*Passiflora incarnata*): mild sedative for insomnia, panic, and seizures.

## Analgesic

In trauma situations and injuries, analgesic herbs are palliative remedies that allow healing to begin while the patient's attention can be drawn elsewhere. Since pain is the body's response to trauma, constant nagging pain is an endless reminder to the patient that something is terribly wrong, and this (sometimes unconscious) realization can lead to insomnia, fear, and anxiety, creating a psychosomatic barrier that delays physical healing. Relieving pain lets the person relax so the body can heal itself.

- **poppy** (*Papaver somniferum*): In ancient times, among the most highly-prized pain killers was opium, the poppy from which we now extract morphine. Doses of opium in tincture form were called laudanum and everyone in the family, including fussy infants, were dosed with this "miracle" medicine. Of course, opium causes severe addictions, but teas and tinctures made with poppy seeds are safe.

- **clove** (*Syzygium aromaticum*): The numbing properties of clove oil are appreciated externally, as long as the oil is very well diluted; just a drop of clove oil in a preparation of salve or ointment can numb the superficial nerves and relieve pain.

## Wound Formulas
### A FORMULA FOR WOUNDS (AS A TINCTURE OR TEA TO DRINK)

› 2 parts lemon balm

› 1 part red clover

› 1 part willow

## A Formula for Wounds (as a salve, compress, or poultice)

› 2 parts elder leaf

› 1 part yarrow

› 1 part red clover

› ½ part comfrey

Be sure to provide plenty of fresh, clean drinking water, since the body tends to "freeze" many of its functions immediately after a trauma, and it will slowly resume these functions once it has perceived the danger is past. For example, digestive function may slow down or temporarily stop, and immediately after such an injury, heart rate and peripheral vascular resistance increase, meaning the heart pumps harder and faster while the blood vessels contract more, leading to a decrease in cardiac output. This prepares the body for an emergency. Slowly, though, approximately twenty-four hours after major burn or other severe laceration injury, cardiac output returns to normal. Drinking water "kick-starts" the body's fluid systems, and consuming vital electrolytes is crucial to maintaining the proper saline balance for bodily fluid systems.

Finally, assisting the person with bandaging, hygiene, and gentle mobility are all important in helping return to a normal, calm, and productive state of being.

## Dry Skin

Dry skin is a common complaint among the elderly, as well as among those who have poor digestive systems, have been taking prescription medications for a long time, or who work in trades where chemical contaminants are the norm. Nobody wants dry skin; it sags, hangs, looks pallid, and is not an effective barrier for keeping the body healthy. Normal healthy skin is supposed to protect the body, retain moisture, and repel germs. Dry skin can harbor germs under scaling cells that continually need to slough off, and its lack of elasticity makes it ill-suited to the job of protection.

Holistic questions include the following: Is she drinking enough water? Is he stressed and exhausted? Is her diet poor, or does she have digestive problems leading to poor nutrient absorption? Is she on high-calcium medication? Or are parasites suspected? It's important to look beneath the surface (literally in this case) to determine the real cause. Most healthy aging people experience supple skin and radiant color, and sagging pallid skin is not the norm.

There are many herbs to call on in support of healthy, well-nourished skin, including nervine tonics (which will be the bulk of the formula in tier 1), emollients, hepatics, cardiac tonics (for better circulation), and digestive aids (especially bitters).

Nervine tonics include those mentioned before, such as lemon balm, motherwort, chamomile, skullcap, red clover, nettle, rhodiola, gotu kola, and passionflower. Motherwort and chamomile are especially useful if high blood pressure is a problem due to anxiety.

Hepatic herbs include dandelion, burdock (especially useful if skin eruptions or acne are a problem), milk thistle, turmeric, and motherwort (these last two are useful if anxiety is an issue).

Cardiac herbs may be useful if blood circulation is not up to par. If the heart cannot pump enough blood at the proper pace, and the blood vessels cannot carry it with the proper strength, then the skin (among other organs) is not getting an adequate supply of oxygen, which can lead to over-dryness. Cardiac toning herbs include hawthorn (good for high blood pressure), prickly ash (useful for increasing circulation to the periphery—such as for cold hands and feet), motherwort (useful for stress, anxiety and tension as well as toning the heart), and linden (a general tonic for hypertension). Other stimulating herbs for the bloodstream, heart, and periphery include ginger, rosemary, and gentian (*Gentiana lutea*), while cayenne and ginkgo strengthen blood flow (to the periphery and head). These indirect support herbs belong in tier 3 or 4 for the skin.

Finally, emollient herbs are soothing, anti-inflammatory moisturizers that help build skin tissue, soothe periphery nerve endings, alleviate itch, and give elasticity and tone. Plant-derived oils such as jojoba, grapeseed, hemp, olive, sweet almond, wheat germ, castor bean, avocado, kukui nut, raspberry seed, and black cumin seed are also emollient. In addition to emollient herbs already discussed, consider rinses or lotions of:

- **rose petal** (*Rosa rugosa*): a light tea or tisane made from the petals can be soothing and very aromatic, calming the nerves.

- **oatstraw** or **oats milky tops** (*Avena sativa*): a creamy lotion can be made from the oats, oat tops or oat straw (stalk) by soaking them in warm water. Strained, this lotion can be applied to dry, itchy skin for fast relief or poured into a bath.

- **jewelweed** (*Impatiens capensis*): the juicy stalk can be rubbed directly onto itchy skin.

### Dry Skin Formulas

#### A FORMULA FOR DRY SKIN (AS A TINCTURE OR TEA TO DRINK)

> › 2 parts nettle
>
> › 1 part passionflower
>
> › 1 part ginger

#### A FORMULA FOR DRY SKIN (AS A SALVE, LOTION, OR OIL)

> › 2 parts calendula
>
> › 1 part rose petal
>
> › 1 part elderflower

# Acne and Skin Eruptions

We all remember our emotionally painful days of adolescence when we were forced to go to school with pimples or zits on our faces. It can be easy to drop a fortune at the nearest pharmacy for over-the-counter or even prescription acne medications. Beyond adolescence, adults can experience acne and skin eruptions for a variety of reasons, including medications, exposure to toxins, liver disease, and stress. Over-the-counter and prescription acne medications seldom work, may disfigure the face even more, contain harsh chemicals that are inhaled and absorbed through the broken lesions, include unnecessary and harmful steroids, and fail to teach our children about the connection between our bodies and Mother Nature.

At puberty, hormones called androgens begin surging forth, those masculinizing hormones that indicate in both sexes that change is underway. Androgens stimulate the sebaceous glands, among others, increasing the volume and thickness of the skin's oil secretions, as well as storing more lipids (fats) in the follicles. Together with emotional ups and downs (which affect the nervous system and the adrenal glands), the teenager's hormonal system seems to launch an assault on the child's skin, resulting in mild acne (a few pimples, blackheads, or whiteheads) or severe acne (spreading pustules, inflamed cysts, and possibly infected sores) across the sebaceous gland areas of the skin: the face, shoulders, upper back, and chest.

For both adolescents and adults, herbal healing addresses the hormonal, nervous, and digestive systems. Anti-inflammatories and topical astringents are useful, and especially lymphatic tonics since they help "drain" fluids from the body and have a strong effect on our core immunity. The treatment for males and females may differ, given the difference in sex hormones, although each sex has the same hormones (estrogen, progesterone, testosterone, androgen) but in varying amounts. Tier 2 Specifics for acne include:

- **burdock** (*Arctium lappa*): use both the leaves and the seeds in tincture form

- **red clover** (*Trifolium pratense*): useful as a tea, tincture, or topical rinse

- **chaste tree berry** (*Vitex agnus-castus*): a pituitary normalizer, chaste tends to balance hormones through the hypothalamus-pituitary axis (HPA).

- **cleavers** (*Galium aparine*): a normalizing alterative herb frequently used for the lymph system, which is indicated in cases of acne for its "flushing" action and its perceived ability to remove toxins from the skin.

- **garlic** (*Allium sativum*): a vital alterative, garlic is used in the treatment of a variety of cardiovascular issues, and here it can be beneficial, as well. Not only is it antibacterial and antifungal, garlic lowers cholesterol in the bloodstream and reduce the built-up lipids of skin.

Emollient herbs soothe the area where scabs have crusted over and the skin needs a moisturizer. Consider calendula, red clover, and chickweed in a light oil such as sunflower or safflower.

- **contraindicated:** Generally, refrain from using mint on acne-affected skin, especially if there are open sores, as mint can sting. Avoid using essential oils (even diluted), since whole-plant medicines (infusions) are far superior for soothing and protecting the delicate skin.

## *Acne and Skin Eruption Formulas*

### A FORMULA FOR ACNE FOR MALES (AS A TINCTURE)

> 2 parts burdock seed

> 1 part red clover

> 1 part cleavers

> ½ part calendula

### A FORMULA FOR ACNE FOR FEMALES (AS A TINCTURE)

> 2 parts burdock seed

> 1 part chaste tree berry

> 1 part cleavers

> ½ part calendula

### A FORMULA FOR ACNE (EXTERNALLY AS A WASH OR RINSE)

> 2 parts calendula

> 1 part red clover

> 1 part chickweed

When using the external wash, rinse with cool water and avoid the eyes.

Because the results are fast and effective, herbal remedies for the skin are well-known and diverse. Our access to strong and safe antimicrobials, antifungals, and antiparasitic herbs, as well as soothing emollients, gives us many options for supporting and assisting the client suffering both acute and chronic issues of the skin.

# PART FIVE

# Hormones and the Endocrine System

Both women and men experience the fluctuations of hormone changes throughout their lives. For women this process is particularly relevant and obvious, but in no instance is hormone change, pregnancy, childbirth, or menopause to be considered an illness. The human body manages these natural processes quite smoothly most of the time; when issues arise, herbs are usually quite capable of rebalancing the body's chemistry and supporting a person's emotional and physical health.

The following chapters offer guidance gleaned from years of personal experience as well as research and study with herbalists from around the country. The topics include menarche (a girl's first period), herbal medicine for women (particularly adult women who can experience reproductive anomalies or symptoms associated with normal menses), pregnancy, childbirth, and post-partum care (offering herbal formulary advise for practitioners of all trades who care for pregnant, laboring and nursing women), and menopause. We'll also look at herbal treatments for two of the more common issues of the endocrine system, specifically for the thyroid and the adrenals. Finally, we'll cover topics of particular interest to men and men's health, including reproductive health, energy, muscle care, and more. The urinary system fits well here and is of interest to both men and women and to any healing arts practitioner interested in keeping a person's digestive system fit and healthy.

# CHAPTER ELEVEN

# Menarche and Herbal Medicine for Teenage Women

Women's use of herbs for physical health dates back millennia; for thousands of years, we have concrete evidence that herbs have been used to heal the human body, and presumably, that includes women's bodies, although many historians have incorrectly presumed "human" simply refers to "men." Women have, undoubtedly, called on plants to heal their wounds, infections, cuts, scrapes, and indigestion, just as men have. But women have special body parts, unique to our gender, that require additional care and tending. The breasts are not just lumps on our chests; they are highly respectable organs with a unique function: providing nourishment to our babies. The uterus is not just a "receptacle" for pregnancy; it is a highly adaptable, flexible organ perfect for attracting the egg, cradling the fetus, squeezing the baby out at the right time, and then resuming its shape. Between babies, the uterus fills with menstrual blood, contains it effectively for twenty-eight days, then expels the blood in an orderly fashion. The ovaries supply essential hormones throughout a woman's life until menopause. Our endocrine system regulates body temperature, emotional balance, water balance, weight gain, and monthly bleeding. The following herbs and formulas are to be used in tandem with the woman's personal experience and, when necessary, with appropriate medical professionals.

Just like with the respiratory system, many of the traditional herbs that form the cornerstone of reproductive herbalism are, sadly, endangered or at-risk. The educational and advocacy organization United Plant Savers has created two lists of herbs that detail which medicinal plants are at-risk or are being watched; the following traditional "women's" herbs are all on the lists (see Glossary E at the back of this book): helonias, or false unicorn root, blue cohosh, black cohosh, beth root (*Trillium*), lady's slipper, wild yam, and partridgeberry.

## Menarche

Menarche is the beginning of the menstrual cycle for a young woman and normally takes place between the ages of ten and sixteen, with twelve being a general average (though every young woman is different). While signs of puberty may begin as early as seven or eight, menarche generally happens later. Menarche is the production of the first egg from its follicle (eggs that have been inside the girl's body since birth), its passage through the uterus, and the first shedding of blood from the uterus. This marks a profound and special time in a girl's life: she is now a woman. Not only has she matured physically and is by nature capable of producing a child of her own, she is also growing into a helpful and thoughtful contributing member of society. This is a time for celebration and honor.

But it can also bring confusion and even fear to the girl who is not prepared to find blood on her underwear. As a facilitator for young women's workshops, I've heard heart-breaking stories of girl's first periods becoming nightmares, and the best antidote to this is proper education from the mother or other trusted adult. Letting girls know what they may soon expect prepares them to think ahead—a strategy they can use the rest of their lives, especially for their periods. Proper planning cultivates body awareness, which includes awareness of ovulation, self-care, body temperature fluctuations, and managing their own contraception when they are ready to become sexually active. Up-front education encourages self-confidence and self-respect. As always, encourage girls to speak freely and share their emotions, thoughts, and symptoms. Also plan to work in tandem with the child's parent and primary care provider since some menstrual symptoms can indicate more serious illnesses.

Herbs can be successful for a variety of conditions, including:

## Anovulation

The absence of ovulation, or egg production, can indicate a number of physiological issues that must be addressed by a health care practitioner, including physical obstruction, hormone imbalance, or other illness. Often herbalists can help coax the person's body into wholeness and rhythm with herbal modulators (also called normalizers) that help bring estrogen and progesterone production into balance. Ovulation is dependent upon an increase in estrogen that stimulates follicle stimulating hormones (FSH), which in turn stimulates the follicle to release an egg. When estrogen fails to rise to necessary levels, FSH will not be stimulated and no egg will be produced. Estrogen levels depend on many factors, of which stress is one. Stress can form on several fronts: over-worked and exhausted women; women who are afraid or who live in fear; women who are very athletic and stress their bodies to the maximum possible; women who are dealing with other hormonal imbalance issues which affect their estrogen and progesterone output; women who experience physical blockages such as fibroids.

Teenagers generally first ovulate between the ages of ten and sixteen (average age twelve), and cycles tend to be sporadic and uneven for at least the first two years after the first cycle. It is not wise to try to stimulate the onset of ovulation and menses through any means; let nature take its course unless there is reason to believe an underlying issue poses a threat to the young woman's health. In fact, most first menstrual cycles are anovulatory, with a full year to a year-and-a-half of a girl's periods producing no eggs. In late onset ovulation, many years can pass before all menstrual cycles involve the production of an egg from the follicle. Educate your female clients about what they may expect with their menstrual cycle, including the fact that it may not be the same every month (duration, saturation, ovulation, and symptoms). However, menstruating women may experience short-term anovulation when, during a cycle, there is no oocyte or egg produced, or they may experience chronic or long-term anovulation which can cause infertility and medical problems such as polycystic ovary syndrome. Menstruation (bleeding) may continue normally despite the lack of ovulation, though light and scant menses occurs in about 40 percent of anovulatory women. Encouraging ovulation (during a normal menstrual cycle) can benefit from any of the following herbal actions:

- **Hormone modulators:** black cohosh (see below), chaste tree berry (see below), wild yam. These increase estrogen in the follicular phase and decrease testosterone, mainly by supporting the adrenal glands.

- **Astrogenic precursor herbs:** red clover

- **Pituitary tonics:** ashwagandha, chaste tree berry

- **Thyroid tonics:** bladderwrack, bugleweed, licorice

- **Adaptogens:** eleuthero, panax ginseng, schisandra, ashwagandha

- **Anxiolytics and nervine tonics:** skullcap, holy basil, oats milky tops, lemon balm, motherwort

- **Mineral-rich herbs:** nettle, alfalfa

- **Bitters:** yarrow, chamomile, motherwort

### *Formulas for Anovulation*
#### A FORMULA FOR ANOVULATION

› 2 parts motherwort

› 1 part red clover

› 1 part nettle

› 1 part chaste tree berry

# Amenorrhea

The absence of menses can have many etiological factors. Primary amenorrhea is diagnosed when there are no periods by age fourteen with no secondary sexual signs of puberty, or by age sixteen regardless of other signs. Secondary amenorrhea is diagnosed when there are no periods for three to six months at any point after menstruation has already begun. Each case can benefit from herbs that balance hormones, though primary amenorrhea can be indicative of more serious underlying problems and merits further investigation by a health care professional. Basic nutrition must be addressed and other factors (such as extreme athleticism or stress) should be considered. For secondary amenorrhea, bitter herbs with emmenagogue or warming effects can prove useful, as well as balancing hormonal herbs. Some tier 2 specific herbs to "bring on" menses include:

- **black cohosh** (*Actaea racemosa*, previously *Cimicifuga racemosa*): Used in seemingly contradictory ways. Traditionally and clinically it has been used to both soothe the uterus and to stimulate it, to prevent miscarriage and also to stimulate the menstrual cycle and childbirth. The Eclectics considered black cohosh an emmenagogue, while contemporary herbalists list it as a relaxing and soothing uterine tonic. All agree that it is useful for painful menses, the "bearing down" feeling of cramps, and to bring on delayed or absent menstruation. Timing is critical for the use of this herb; to use it for delayed menses is to use it as a stimulant; to use it to strengthen uterine contractions for childbirth is to use it as a stimulant; however, to use it during menstruation is to use it as a relaxing antispasmodic.

- **ginger** (*Zingiber officinale*): As a warming and diaphoretic herb, ginger gets blood moving. It's highly useful as a women's herb for pelvic congestion and delayed menses. It can be taken as a hot infusion, or as a tincture, or used topically as a warm compress on the lower abdomen to stimulate decongestion and relieve pain.

- **chaste tree berry** (*Vitex agnus castus*): the berries were used by European monks to suppress their libido, earning them the name "chaste tree berries." But modern women often enhance the libido, indicating the herb is a pituitary normalizer. Vitex is commonly employed to normalize a menstrual cycle when the onset is uneven, delayed, or too soon (oligomenorrhea or poly-menorrhea).

- **dong quai** (*Angelica sinensis*): generally used as an emmenagogue and uterine tonic, demonstrating both stimulating and relaxing actions. It is anti-inflammatory, antispasmodic, and analgesic, making it a reliable remedy for many menstrual issues including dysmenorrhea, endometriosis, fibroids, surgical convalescence, and amenorrhea. Another contradictory herb, angelica is used as a calming uterine pregnancy tonic in Traditional Chinese Medicine, whereas in Western herbalism it is avoided during pregnancy. The root is used medicinally while the seeds and stem are sometimes candied.

- **mugwort** (*Artemisia vulgaris*): strong and bitter, this is a warming emmenagogue.

- **yarrow** (*Achillea millefolium*): also contradictory. Yarrow is generally used as a diaphoretic, warming, stimulating, and yet astringent herb. But in many uterine and menstrual disorders, it can achieve relaxing effects that can bewilder a beginning herbalist. For delayed menses, a strong cup of hot yarrow infusion can stimulate the uterus to contract.

- **cinnamon** (*Cinnamomum* spp.): Used as a warming stimulant, small doses of cinnamon can bring on delayed menses. However, amenorrhea that is due to pituitary or other endocrine issues, hormonal imbalances, or physical obstruction will not benefit from this herb. Cinnamon can be taken with food (the best way) or carefully infused into an oil for a warm external application. Caution: many people find cinnamon irritating to the skin, so this method should be used with care and in limited doses.

## *Amenorrhea Formulas*

### A FORMULA FOR PRIMARY AMENORRHEA (AS A TEA, TINCTURE, OR CAPSULE)

› 2 parts licorice

› 2 part black cohosh

› 2 parts chaste tree berry

› 1 part raspberry leaf

### A FORMULA FOR SECONDARY AMENORRHEA

› 2 parts chamomile

› 1 part dong quai

› 1 part yarrow

› 1 part nettle

# Dysmenorrhea

Dysmenorrhea is painful menses, including cramps, a "pulling down" feeling in the vagina, often accompanied by headache, dizziness, sweats, irritability, and either constipation or diarrhea. Herbalists generally work symptomatically and use herbs as a nourishing foundation, as well as providing herbs that are anti-spasmodic, anti-inflammatory, warming, and anodyne. Tier 2 Specifics for painful menses include:

- **wild yam** (*Dioscorea villosa*): taken as an infusion or tincture, this is one of the most reliable herbs for pelvic inflammation, uterine congestion, and pelvic pain. The wild yam-derived "pill" has been used in allopathic medicine to remedy this condition effectively, but with considerable side effects. Wild yam is especially helpful in cases where the downward pull sensation (the heavy pull) in the vagina is persistent and energy-depleting.

- **ginger** (*Zingiber officinale*): warming and diaphoretic, the tea stimulates blood circulation throughout the body. Can also be used as a compress over the abdomen.

- **helonias** (*Chamaelirium luteum*): false unicorn root or helonias is an herb with contradictory uses, sometimes being used as an anti-inflammatory and relaxant, while at other times serving as an emmenagogue and stimulant. Habitat loss and overharvesting threaten this plant and it is listed on the United Plant Savers (UpS) at-risk list (see Glossary E).

- **raspberry** (*Rubus ideaus*): As a uterine tonic and strengthener, raspberry can help in cases where the pain is due to atony or insufficient tone, where the uterus is weak, where pelvic muscles are weak, or where there is a nutrient deficit.

General anodynes that could be placed in tier 3 of a formula for pelvic pain include meadowsweet, willow, and Jamaican dogwood. Meadowsweet and willow, in my experience, truly benefit from the presence of a vehicle herb that will carry them to the desired location in the body. I've found they respond well to feverfew and ginkgo in the treatment of headaches, and to raspberry and wild yam in the treatment of painful menses and cramps. Jamaican dogwood is renowned as a muscle relaxer and muscle-pain reliever, particularly useful for nighttime cramps and insomnia.

Warming herbs can help both internally and externally and can be placed in the tier 3 of a formula for pelvic pain. Ginger can assist where dysmenorrhea causes nausea and dizziness, and externally it provides a warming compress over the lower abdomen to help reduce spasms and cramps. Yarrow can help eliminate pelvic congestion but both yarrow and ginger can be too stimulating in certain cases; some women find cooling herbs more helpful in "taming" the fire of menstruation. Cooling herbs such as chickweed, lavender and skullcap can be drunk as teas or soaked in cool cloths for external fomentations. Peppermint is generally more warming, while spearmint is more cooling.

Antispasmodics (to reduce muscle spasm and cramps) of primary importance to the pelvis include black haw (*Viburnum prunifolium*) and cramp bark (*Viburnum opulus*) and Jamaican dogwood.

Stress can aggravate the symptoms of dysmenorrhea, causing headaches, shoulder and neck tension, nosebleeds, nausea, and depression. Consider passionflower, chamomile, skullcap, and vervain (see Calming and Nervine Herbs in chapter 6).

*Dysmenorrhea Formulas*

### A FORMULA FOR DYSMENORRHEA, UTERINE CONGESTION, AND MENSTRUAL PAIN

> › 2 parts chamomile

> › 1 part wild yam

> › 1 part ginger

> › 1 part Jamaican dogwood

### ANOTHER FORMULA FOR DYSMENORRHEA, UTERINE CONGESTION, AND MENSTRUAL PAIN

> › 2 parts cramp bark

> › 1 part wild yam

> › 1 part chaste tree berry

> › 1 part passionflower

## Menorrhagia, Metrorragia, and Anemia

The over-production and over-expulsion of menstrual blood from the uterus is menorrhagia, and is often caused by low blood levels of progesterone. Menorrhagic women experience a very high level of menstrual blood which often occurs over a longer period of time than normal menstrual cycles. Though normal varies per person, most women spend three to six days menstruating and lose thirty to eighty milliliters of blood, or approximately two to four tampons. Excess menstrual blood loss can lead to fatigue, mineral loss, uterine atony, and anemia. Metrorrhagia is irregular heavy bleeding.

Hormonal balancing herbs can help (the best include wild yam, chaste tree berry, and black cohosh), as well as pituitary and adrenal tonic herbs such as licorice or lemon balm.

Antispasmodics can reduce symptomatic cramping and possibly reduce blood loss; cramp bark (*Viburnum opulus*), black haw (*Viburnum prunifolium*), black cohosh, and wild yam are key possibilities. Motherwort

(*Leonurus cardiaca*) and spearmint (*Mentha spicata*) are anti-inflammatory, aiding the body in its efforts to relax.

Astringents can help stem the tide of blood flowing and help the body reabsorb critical minerals instead of expelling them. Key astringent herbs for the uterus include shepherd's purse, lady's mantle (*Alchemilla mollis, A. vulgaris*), partridgeberry (*Mitchella repens*) and cranesbill (*Geranium maculatum*). Here, yarrow displays its contradictory nature; though normally warming and stimulating when drunk hot (and used as a classic emmenagogue to bring on menses), some herbalists use it for its astringency to curb excessive bleeding. In this case, use yarrow as a douche or drink it as a cold infusion.

Because menorrhagic women lose more blood than normally menstruating women, they are at greater risk for iron depletion and anemia. Symptoms of anemia include shortness of breath (especially during and after exertion), fatigue, dizziness, headaches, pale skin, and rapid heart rate and/or chest pains. Eating and taking iron-rich and folic acid–rich herbs can greatly benefit women's endocrine system, skin, hair, nails, liver, and digestive systems. Iron-rich herbs include amaranth, dried apricots, bladderwrack, chlorella, dandelion leaf and root, dates, kelp, lamb's quarters, licorice, pumpkin seeds, blackstrap molasses, mustard greens, nettle, oatstraw, and bran, parsley, prunes, raisins, sarsaparilla, thyme, watercress, and yellow dock. Take iron-rich foods alongside bitters or foods high in vitamin C, such as oranges or citrus fruits. Avoid alcohol and coffee, which sap iron from the body. Soy should be eaten separately.

### Menorrhagia, Metrorrhagia, and Anemia Formulas
#### A Formula for Menorrhagia
  › 2 parts motherwort

  › 1 part wild yam

  › 1 part shepherd's purse

  › 1 part partridgeberry

### A Formula for Anemia

> › 2 parts nettle

> › 1 part dandelion root

> › 1 part oats milky tops

> › 1 part yellow dock root

### Another Formula for Anemia (as a syrup)

To make the syrup, simmer the nettle, dates and apricots in enough water to cover for 15 minutes. Strain and add molasses to desired thickness. Refrigerate and take by the tablespoonful.

> › 2 parts nettle

> › 3 to 5 dates, pitted

> › 5 to 7 dried apricots, chopped

> › 2 parts molasses

## Growing Bones

Growing women have growing bones; they are not only a uterus, but an entire body! The teenage years are prime years for adding length and support to the skeletal structure. Be sure teenage women get plenty of calcium, as this necessary mineral contributes not only to bones and teeth but also to muscle control, nerve function, proper glandular secretion, blood clotting, and to future prevention of osteoporosis.

To maintain strong bones, encourage girls and women to indulge in the mineral-rich herbs listed here as well as foods that promote proper calcium absorption. Eat dairy products (especially yogurt), meat as desired, some seafood (especially oysters and sardines), and lots of beet greens and beans. Calcium is best absorbed along with sufficient vitamin D (sunlight exposure and vitamin-D fortified milk are best) and vitamin C. Avoid sodas with calcium-rich foods; the phosphorus that contributes to the carbonation can interfere with calcium absorption. A healthy infusion can be made by combining fennel seeds, poppy seeds, dried raspberry leaves, and dried nettle leaves, or a lightly salty snack can be made by combining mineral-rich sesame seeds, celery seeds, dill seeds, and fennel seeds. The following herbs are high in minerals:

- **horsetail** (*Equisetum arvense*): Horsetail is high in silica, calcium, magnesium, chromium, potassium, iron, and copper, and also rich in bioflavonoids and carotenoids

- **oats** (*Avena sativa*): Also called oats milky tops. Encourage teens to eat oatmeal for breakfast (raw or cooked), as well as in oat snacks such as granola, oat-and-millet balls, and trail mix. Oats supply vitamins, calcium, magnesium, chromium, and silica.

### Bones Support Formulas
#### A FORMULA FOR BONE SUPPORT

› 2 parts oats milky tops

› 2 parts alfalfa

› 1 part horsetail

› 1 part nettle

## Depression

The onset of menses can bring about profound emotional changes, and coupled with normal life stress, these changes can produce feelings of depression, uncertainty, abandonment, hopelessness, and anger. Girls experiencing these feelings should be cared for with respect and compassion; severe depression requires immediate emergency response. For mild depression and hormonal swings, see Chapter 6.

# Acne

A maddening and embarrassing skin condition, acne is usually the result of hormone imbalance, especially from the pituitary gland. Teens and adults suffering from acne can develop mild to disfiguring sores, pustules, boils, abscesses, and even long-term scarring.

Many herbalists use alterative herbs for internal balancing to realign the endocrine system and clear the skin from the inside out. Supporting and strengthening the lymphatic and hepatic systems are key in helping the body expel toxins and metabolic wastes through the proper channels. As mentioned earlier, herbs of particular importance in this process are chaste tree, dandelion leaf and root, and red clover, while others indicated in acne include yellow dock root, cleavers, and milk thistle. Externally, compresses and facial astringents can be made from astringent and emollient herbs such as witch hazel, calendula, burdock root, burdock seed, lavender, and mullein. These soothing and cooling herbs help clear the skin, reduce inflammation and heat, cool the face and neck, and tighten tissues.

## Acne Formulas

### A FORMULA FOR HORMONE-BASED ACNE (AS A TEA, TINCTURE, OR CAPSULE)

› 2 parts chaste tree berry

› 2 parts red clover

› 1 part dandelion leaf

› 1 part cleavers

### ANOTHER FORMULA FOR ACNE (AS A WASH OR COMPRESS)

› 2 parts witch hazel

› 2 parts calendula

› 1 part mullein leaf

# Bloating

Bloating is a common symptom during menstruation and typically goes away when bleeding ends. Be sure to distinguish common bloating from the more serious issue of fibroids, which can produce somewhat similar symptoms but are rare in women under age twenty (see next chapter). Pelvic congestion during menstruation often responds well to wild yam, black cohosh, and ginger, as these are anti-spasmodic and anti-inflammatory herbs with a special affinity for the uterus. Warming carminative herbs can also be very helpful: caraway, dill, fennel, chamomile, motherwort, lemon balm, lavender, and mint. Cramp bark and black haw can be effective antispasmodics to reduce spastic irritation in the uterus and pelvic area.

## *Bloating Formulas*
### A FORMULA FOR BLOATING (AS A TINCTURE OR TEA TO DRINK)

> › 2 parts spearmint
> › 2 parts chamomile
> › 1 part wild yam
> › 1 part cramp bark

Supporting the young woman as she grows from a girl to an adult is a privilege we cannot take for granted. Introducing young women to the beauty and power of herbal medicines has been one of the rich joys of my herbal career, and it is so worthwhile to freely share our knowledge and heritage with the young people who will take over our traditions. Because the endocrine system is so delicate, especially during adolescence, be sure to work in tandem with other health care providers to develop a well-rounded approach to support the natural occurrences of menarche and menstruation.

# CHAPTER TWELVE

# Herbal Medicine for Midlife Women

Throughout her menstruating life, a woman will experience highs and lows of estrogen, progesterone, luteinizing hormone, and follicle stimulating hormone. Though perfectly natural and normal, these cycles can sometimes contribute to imbalances that present as pre-menstrual syndrome (also called pre-menstrual tension) or that can lead to infertility.

## Pre-Menstrual Syndrome (or Pre-Menstrual Tension)

Women's hormones are an extremely complex system of the human body and, to date, not much is known about them. Science has pinpointed the provenance of certain hormone production—identifying particular organs in the body as manufacturing and distribution points—and it has a good handle on the general menstrual cycle and even a woman's hormonal cycle throughout her lifetime. But science doesn't understand a great deal about the particulars of how tender hormones act, why they affect the emotions, or how they instigate weight gain, etc. What about painful menses? Or the absence of menses? It can take years of careful observation for a young healthy woman to determine why she's anovulatory, for example. Medical science hasn't pinpointed how stress affects hormonal balance, how to accurately gauge the amount of progesterone or estrogen in the body at a particular time, whether skin eruptions are the result of changing hormones, or how diet affects the chemical reaction of hormones in the female body.

We need to know the herbal answers to these questions. We are gaining ground, especially since herbalists look at the body holistically and take into consideration issues that are often ignored by medical science, such as stress, diet, and environmental factors.

Mild pre-menstrual syndrome appears to affect 40 percent of women of reproductive age, with 85 percent of women reporting at least one symptom each month. Moderate to debilitating PMS affects about 3 percent. Debilitating symptoms include severe anger, anxiety, mood swings and depression—enough that daily life ceases to function normally; this is referred to as pre-menstrual dysphoric disorder (PMDD).

Women often experience a conglomerate of symptoms during the late luteal phase of the cycle: headaches, fatigue, emotional duress, anxiety, fluid retention, sore and swollen breasts, acne, nosebleeds, confusion, insomnia, and many more common physical and emotional symptoms associated with a drop in estrogen and a spike in progesterone. Just before the period begins, progesterone plunges. Many women experience a reduction or elimination of symptoms once bleeding begins, or within a day or two of menses.

## Herbal Actions for PMS

The following conditions can be alleviated by the appropriate herbal actions:

## Hormone Imbalance

Balancing the varying levels of estrogen and progesterone is the job of the tier 2 specific:

- **chaste tree berry** (*Vitex agnus-castus*): taken regularly throughout the entire menstrual cycle, chaste tree berry acts as a hormonal modulator, most likely through its influence on the hypothalamus-pituitary-adrenal (HPA) axis and its apparent effects as a pituitary normalizer. The berries contain essential oils and flavonoids and can reduce follicle-stimulating hormone (FSH) levels and increase luteinizing hormone (LH) levels. This balancing can result in decreased estrogen and increased progesterone.

- **black cohosh** (*Actaea racemosa*): valued for the hot flashes of perimenopause and as a hormone modulator helpful for PMS. Romm lists it as useful for PMS with headache;[70] Hoffmann lists is as a "normalizer" and relaxant.[71] Black cohosh seems to have no direct effect on hormone production and contains no hormone precursors; it is used as an antispasmodic and muscle relaxant with a special affinity for the uterus with the peculiar ability to both relax smooth muscle contractions (ease cramps) and to stimulate smooth muscle contractions (aiding in childbirth). Use as a tonic to maintain uterine tone. For PMS its most outstanding features are cramp relief, headache relief, and as a nervine tonic, helpful for hormone-induced depression and anxiety.

---

70    Romm (2010).

71    Hoffmann (1996).

### Inflammation of the Pelvic Area

Herbs that relieve pelvic congestion and inflammation of the uterus can help with cramping, bloating, gas, diarrhea, pain, dysmenorrhea, and PMS symptoms. Consider wild yam, black cohosh, licorice, and motherwort.

### Emotional Irritability

If emotional extremism is the key issue the woman is experiencing, use motherwort, skullcap, and black cohosh as tier 2 Specifics; otherwise consider them tier 1 tonics.

### Breast Tenderness and Swelling

Caused by fluid retention, believed to be caused by increased aldosterone levels, breast tenderness is a noncritical symptom of PMS that causes discomfort. Sodium intake can aggravate breast tenderness and increase the risk of cardiovascular problems. In addition to the diuretic herbs dandelion and parsley for edema and PMS-related swelling, consider:

- **evening primrose** (*Oenothera biennis*): the oil extracted from the seed is an effective agent for the support of pain-free breasts, boasting a high content of gamma-linolenic acid (GLA), a soothing fatty acid that relieves exhausted bodies from having to manufacture the acid themselves. Humans normally manufacture GLA from linoleic acid, a metabolic process necessary when we eat food such as sunflower seeds. But the metabolism creates waste in the body, much like an automobile breaking down gasoline creates exhaust. Evening primrose gives our bodies the pure, unadulterated fatty acid it needs, without any conversion necessary, reducing the stress our bodies experience during the luteal phase of menstruation.

*PMS Forumlas*

### A FORMULA FOR PMS WITH BREAST TENDERNESS (AS A TINCTURE OR TEA)

› 2 parts oats milky tops

› 1 part dandelion leaf

› 1 part dandelion root

› additional support: evening primrose oil capsules

### A FORMULA FOR PMS WITH HEADACHE (AS A TINCTURE OR TEA)

› 2 parts lemon balm

› 1 part motherwort

› 1 part black haw

› 1 part feverfew

› 1 part ginkgo

### A FORMULA FOR PMS WITH MOOD SWINGS (AS A TINCTURE OR TEA)

› 2 parts motherwort

› 1 part lemon balm

› 1 part skullcap

› 1 part gotu kola

› additional support: magnesium supplement

## Fibroids

Among the most common issues a woman faces (approximately half of all women will develop one or more fibroids by age fifty, with African and African-American women more susceptible than Caucasian), these noncancerous tumors are nevertheless important to understand as they can cause side effects such as bloating, pain, heavy bleeding (menorrhagia), and in-between bleeding (metrorrhagia). Fibroids are suspected to be caused by excess estrogen and they can range in size from microscopic to as large as the entire uterus, requiring surgery.

Symptoms associated with fibroids include heavy bleeding and bleeding between periods, extended length of menses, excessive urination or the urge to urinate, pelvic cramping, pelvic fullness or congestion, pain, and/or pain during intercourse. Treatment for fibroids can involve doing nothing (most fibroids shrink and disappear at the onset of menopause or they may be so small that they cause no symptoms) to surgery, as well as treatment for corollary symptoms such as pain, swelling (edema), lethargy, the sensation of fullness, and anemia.

Herbal treatment for fibroids focuses on hormone modulators that balance the levels of estrogen and progesterone in the blood. The best tier 2 specific is chaste tree berry (*Vitex agnus-castus*). Tier 3 and tier 4 symptomatic support comes from:

- **Astringents:** lady's mantle, shepherd's purse, yarrow, cranesbill, raspberry leaf

- **Antispasmodics:** black haw, cramp bark, skullcap

- **Anti-inflammatories:** evening primrose oil, borage seed oil, black currant seed oil, safflower seed oil, hemp seed oil, spirulina

- **Uterine decongestants:** wild yam

- **Nervine tonics:** skullcap, passionflower, vervain, lemon balm, motherwort

- **Uterine tonics:** raspberry leaf, black cohosh, wild yam

- **Anodynes:** meadowsweet, willow, Jamaican dogwood

Because fibroids cause excessive bleeding, anemia can be an issue. Symptoms of anemia include shortness of breath (especially during and after exertion), fatigue, dizziness, headaches, pale skin, and rapid heart rate, and/or chest pains. Eating and taking iron-rich and folic-acid rich herbs can greatly benefit women's endocrine system, skin, hair, nails, liver, and digestive systems and can replenish iron lost during heavy menses. Animal meats provide both heme and non-heme iron while plant sources provide non-heme, which is slightly less bioavailable than heme.

## Iron-Rich Herbs and Foods

| | | |
|---|---|---|
| amaranth | dried apricots | bladderwrack & kelp |
| dandelion leaf and root | dates | lamb's quarters |
| licorice | pumpkin seeds | blackstrap molasses |
| mustard greens | nettles | oatstraw |
| parsley | prunes | raisins |
| sarsaparilla | watercress | thyme |
| yellow dock | lentils, beans and chickpeas | chocolate |
| oysters and seafoods (heme) | red and white meats (heme) | |

Take iron-rich foods alongside bitters or vitamin C foods, such as oranges or citrus fruits. Avoid alcohol and coffee, which sap iron from the body. Soy should be eaten separately. Include bitters when eating iron-rich foods to aid in absorption. For instance, consuming iron-rich dandelion roots along with bitter dandelion greens is an ideal way to get balanced nutrition. Other bitters include motherwort (in limited quantities during pregnancy), chamomile, green tea, and mustard greens.

Though fibroids that cause pain and other symptoms should be evaluated by a health care provider, these formulas provide support and secondary symptomatic relief in addition to a healthy diet and careful monitoring by a professional.

*Fibroid Formulas*

### A FORMULA FOR FIBROIDS WITH EDEMA

> › 2 parts dandelion leaf
>
> › 1 part raspberry leaf
>
> › 1 part lady's mantle
>
> › 1 part cleavers

### A FORMULA FOR FIBROIDS WITH PAIN

> › 2 parts motherwort
>
> › 2 parts wild yam
>
> › 1 part Jamaican dogwood or turmeric
>
> › 1 part meadowsweet

### A FORMULA FOR FIBROIDS WITH HEAVY BLEEDING

> › 2 parts nettle
>
> › 2 parts wild yam
>
> › 1 part shepherd's purse
>
> › 1 part chaste tree berry

## Fertility

Infertility is diagnosed when a couple has unsuccessfully attempted to conceive for twelve months. Nine out of ten couples successfully conceive in this timeframe, so that absence of success indicates imbalances in either the man or the woman. These imbalances can come from a wide range of causes, including ovulatory disorders (defects in the ovaries or the lack of ovulation), thyroid disorders, adrenal insufficiency, pelvic infection or inflammation, and (rarely) sperm antibodies in the vaginal mucus. Stress is a large contributor to infertility, creating a self-inflicting cycle where more stress creates more infertile months that create more stress.

Careful work with a health care practitioner to rule out physical illness is especially important so that appropriate remedies can be given. Again, black cohosh and chaste tree berry are tier 2 Specifics, which raises concerns of over-harvesting for black cohosh. Though black cohosh contains no estrogen-like compounds itself, it has clinically demonstrated estrogen-modulating activity and the ability to reduce elevated LH levels while not affecting FSH and prolactin. [72]

This makes it useful for infertility derived from anovulation and amenorrhea. Chaste tree's positive effects on balancing the pituitary gland make it valuable in cases of metrorrhagia (bleeding between cycles), polymenorrhea (too frequent cycles), and oligomenorrhea (too few cycles).

Nervine tonics and anxiolytics are key herbs for infertility treatment due to the effects of stress and anxiety. Consider oats, lemon balm, motherwort (but cease motherwort as soon as pregnancy begins), passionflower, skullcap, verbena, and St. John's wort. Ashwagandha is a wonderfully supportive herb in that it will provide a strong basis from which the body can exert its energies for conception.

I don't recommend aphrodisiac herbs, such as damiana, for fertility, except to enhance energy and give the woman a sense of vigor and self-confidence. Combining damiana with roses, clove, vanilla, chocolate, and/or gotu kola can be a fun way to boost arousal and create in-the-moment awareness in anticipation of making love. But long-term efforts that involve hormone balancing and nervous system support should form the foundation of the formula.

---

72   Romm (2010), 339.

*Fertility Formulas*
### A FORMULA FOR INFERTILITY

> › 2 parts chaste tree berry

> › 1 part passionflower

> › 1 part black cohosh

> › 1 part ashwagandha

For women who have been menstruating for years, herbs are a natural choice for supporting their health and addressing the more common imbalances that can occur. This is a prime opportunity to use tonics and to introduce women to the mineral-rich and nourishing herbs that they can rely on long-term.

# CHAPTER THIRTEEN

# Pregnancy, Childbirth, and Post-partum Care

One of the true life-changing phases of a woman's life cycle, pregnancy brings ups and downs, physical changes, emotional challenges, and unimaginable blessings. While many women experience pregnancy without any complications and give birth quickly and easily, other women experience some normal side effects from hormonal changes, or their labors may be difficult for unseen reasons. Supporting the woman and her body, mind and spirit through this transitional time is paramount for the health of mother, father, baby, and siblings. Herbs are the natural supporters to help nourish the body, ease the emotions, and heal illnesses.

Because there are many comprehensive books about herbal remedies for pregnancy, this chapter will be a broad-spectrum introduction to creating herbal formulas for pregnancy, childbirth, and post-partum.

# Pregnancy

Professional midwives have long been the go-to experts for information and education about the application of herbal medicine for pregnancy and childbirth. Midwives provide gynecologic and obstetric care even for women pre-conception, and they are often well-versed in how a woman's body reacts and responds to plant medicines. Pregnancy is not an illness; it is a normal function of a woman's body that has evolved to carry out this part of the life cycle with strength and vigor. However, just like in the cardiovascular or digestive systems, normal processes are impeded by poor nutrition, environmental or genetic factors, or stressful conditions that put the body's systems at a disadvantage.

## Mineral Supplementation

The baby receives most of its nutrition through the umbilicus and feeds off the food the mother ingests. However, if the diet is lacking or if the mother is low on nutrients, the mother's body becomes a donation center providing needed minerals for the baby's growth. This depletion affects the mother's body now as well as in the future, putting her at risk for osteoporosis.

### Herbs and Foods High in Calcium

| | | |
|---|---|---|
| raspberry leaf | nettle | oatstraw and milky tops |
| horsetail | lamb's quarters | fennel seeds |
| sesame seeds | yogurt | cheese and milk |
| fresh steamed greens | whole grains | lentils, beans, and chickpeas |

Include vitamin C rich–foods along with calcium-rich foods to aid in absorption, and avoid drinking sodas and even carbonated waters during pregnancy since the phosphorous that contributes to the carbonation can interfere with calcium absorption. Other mineral-rich herbs include red clover, alfalfa, chamomile, and violet leaves, all of which can be brewed together or separately to make healing and nutrient-packed infusions.

Another important mineral for pregnancy is iron; for sources of iron, see the table "iron-rich herbs and foods."

## Morning Sickness

Morning sickness or nausea is a common symptom of pregnancy and is truly misnamed—it lasts not only through the morning but often all day. Most women experience relief of nausea by the second trimester of pregnancy. Causes are believed to include low blood sugar, low hydrochloric acid, vitamin B6 deficiency, and increased levels of hormones in the bloodstream.

Encourage your clients to prepare snacks at the bedside table and eat before even getting out of bed. Also, eating during the night can help keep foods and fluids in the digestive system so that upon arising in the morning, the body does not feel empty and blood sugar levels do not plummet. Suitable foods for the morning include plain crackers, crackers with peanut or almond butter, tiny strips of dry, non-greasy bacon or jerky, celery with nut butters, dried fruit, candied ginger, popcorn, dried seaweed, and toast. Calcium-rich yogurt is also a good standby for early morning eating.

Herbs that have traditionally shown promise and efficacy in treating morning sickness include wild yam, mint and ginger. Wild yam (not the sweet potato) is the famous root of the South American vine that is the source of the pill. Wild yam balances hormonal production, tones the liver, is anti-inflammatory, especially for the pelvic region, and can be used in cases of premenstrual syndrome to great effect. During pregnancy, wild yam can be a useful remedy for nausea, and it combines well with the tart-tasting dong quai (*Angelica sinensis* or *A. archangelica*) or the bland-tasting chaste tree berry (*Vitex agnus-castus*), which can help balance estrogen and progesterone.

Mint has long been a staple in the medicine cabinet for nausea. Peppermint, spearmint, lemon balm, and catnip are all in the *Lamiaceae* family and are useful for dispelling gas and improving digestive and gastrointestinal function. They are also very useful for the pregnant woman seeking a soothing, calming, and nervine effect in addition to a nausea medication. Mint-family herbs in teas can all help; here are the differences between them:

- **peppermint** (*Mentha × piperita)*: Peppermint is a strong mint with a vasodilating and warming effect on the body. Traditionally used to ease nausea and spasms in the gut, peppermint can be too strong for women who have miscarried or are at risk for miscarriage, as it can act as an emmenagogue in certain cases.

- **spearmint** (*Mentha spicata)*: spearmint is milder and has a sweeter aroma and flavor than the more pungent and biting peppermint. Spearmint is used for digestive disturbances, indigestion, gas, bloating, and nervous issues including nervous exhaustion and anxiety. This is a good choice for the woman who can't tolerate peppermint or who is suffering nausea as a result of stress or nervous tension.

- **lemon balm** (*Melissa officinalis)*: A true nervine tonic, lemon balm shares many characteristics with its mint relatives that make it an ideal morning sickness remedy. It is at once relaxing and invigorating, helping to restore energy and vitality to a woman experiencing fatigue, lethargy, or even mild depression and frustration with her pregnancy. As a carminative, lemon balm eases gas pains, nausea, bloating, and hunger pains; it is strongly nervine and helps stimulate blood flow to the central nervous system to alleviate exhaustion, forgetfulness, confusion, anxiety, and fear. Many women rely on lemon balm in the last stages of pregnancy when "mental fog" sets in and a sense of fear and concern about delivery makes her anxious.

- **catnip** (*Nepeta cataria*): Similar to spearmint, small amounts of catnip can be taken to ease morning sickness. It offers a slight sedative action and is safe for children; it combines well with chamomile. A good remedy for women who are nervous to the point of irritability and whose nausea makes them cranky and upset, and for insomnia.

Make teas of these herbs in small quantities that can be sipped at less-than-acute symptom dosage since their effects on the individual can vary widely. These herbs can also be made into ice cubes to be sucked on, or into concentrated tinctures (dose: ¼ teaspoon every 15–30 minutes until symptoms subside).

# Childbirth

Parturition, or delivery, is the event of the baby leaving the mother's body. It's a powerful transition from pregnancy to the new experience of motherhood, involving a number of issues on both physical and emotional levels.

## Supporting Uterine Contractions

At the onset of labor, a number of stimulant herbs have been traditionally used to "induce" the uterus to begin contractions. All throughout the pregnancy, stimulating herbs have been avoided, but now is the time to use them if they are required. These herbs help activate uterine muscle contraction and open the cervix for passage of the baby's head. Traditional uterine stimulants for delivery include helonias (false unicorn root, *Chamaelirium luteum*), blue cohosh (*Caulophyllum thalictroides*), and black cohosh (*Actaea racemosa*,). All three of these herbs are on the UpS lists (see Glossary E); acceptable substitutes include ginger (*Zingiber officinale*), peppermint (*Mentha ×piperita*). These can be taken as homeopathic tablets or as herbal infusions and tinctures, with 5 to 20 drops given every 15 to 20 minutes until contractions are steady, rhythmic, and strong.

### Labia preparation

Many women fear the stretching and tearing of the vagina and labia; teaching them to moisturize, stretch, and prepare these tissues can alleviate their fears and reduce the need for episiotomies. The best way to prepare these tissues is to maintain a proper diet throughout pregnancy, to keep hydrated, and to consume omega-3 fatty acid foods. Dry tissues don't stretch. But for women whose fear of tearing directly hinders her emotional and physical ability to progress through labor, the application of emollient herbal remedies can be the difference between a frightening, painful process and a peaceful delivery. The best methods for moisturizing labia tissues include gently rubbing with an oil infused with mallow, calendula, red clover, or plantain, or with the oil (fresh or from a broken capsule) of evening primrose. This can be repeated throughout labor, if desired.

### Transition

Midwives view transition as a perfectly normal part of labor that indicates passage from the active stage of labor to the pushing stage. Transition could aptly be named Supreme Panic or The Changing of the Mind. It is a pivotal stage of labor in which the cervix opens completely and the uterus ends "massage" contractions and begins "expulsion" contractions. Transition has a strong impact on the emotions, causing panic, fear, heightened anxiety, uncertainty, and even anger. But it is the shortest stage of labor, lasting only a few minutes to no more than two hours.

Because transition is such a short phase and it is completely normal, it is rarely medicated. But if the mother is truly frightened, angry, anxious, and confused, it is perfectly safe to soothe her with words, massage, and nervine tonics. Tier 1 and 2 nervine tonics and adaptogens bring the body into a state of emotional balance without being sedative; the best are skullcap (*Scutellaria lateriflora*), black cohosh (*Actaea racemosa*), passionflower (*Passiflora incarnata*), and motherwort (*Leonurus cardiaca*). Nervines with a notable sedative action include hops (*Humulus lupulus*) and valerian (*Valeriana officinalis*).

## Hydration

Keeping the body hydrated is an important and sometimes tricky concern during childbirth, as excess pressure on the kidneys and bladder is unwanted though the body must have a continual supply of water. Often the best method for hydrating the mother is to provide frozen chips of water. Frozen chips of raspberry infusion are valuable as these provide a little flavor and the tonic action of raspberry leaf. Keeping the lips protected with a beeswax-based salve is also a good strategy for helping women avoid the "dry lips" feeling of dehydration, making sure the woman has ready access to fresh liquids in addition to use of the ointment.

## Tears and Episiotomies: Post-Partum Tissue Care

Caring for vaginal and labial tears is a common practice for midwives and herbalists, and these wounds can be considered normal events for most childbirths. Extreme wounds that require excessive suturing or demonstrate infection should be seen by a health care practitioner. Herbal formulas should include oils with styptic, vulnerary, antimicrobial, emollient, and astringent actions—all to be used externally only, as most of these are not suitable to the newly breastfeeding mother.

## Emollient and Vulnerary Herbs for Post-Partum Tissue Care

| | | |
|---|---|---|
| raspberry leaf | comfrey leaf | mallow root or leaf |
| calendula | red clover | plantain |
| sage | witch hazel | oak bark |
| lady's mantle | shepherd's purse | St. John's wort |
| yarrow | peppermint | elder leaf or flower |

A combination of any of these herbs can be applied externally as an oil and/or a sitz bath using the following guidelines:

- **Vulnerary oils** are made by infusing the (preferably fresh) chopped plant material in a clean oil such as olive or sweet almond. This preparation should be made weeks in advance, or it can be made quickly by infusing the herbs into the oil on the stovetop over very low heat for twenty to thirty minutes. Strain the herbs carefully through muslin cloth so as not to introduce any fibrous residue to the healing tissues. With a clean cotton ball, swab the oils onto the labia to keep them moisturized, clean, and pliable.

- **A sitz bath** is a strong tea or infusion made with (preferably dried) herbs infused in just-boiled water. The herbs can steep fifteen to twenty minutes or for several hours, even overnight. The taste is irrelevant, but it is essential to extract as much astringency from the herbs as possible. Strain carefully using a muslin cloth and warm the infusion to body temperature or slightly warmer. Pour into a sitz bath tray (available at the pharmacy) positioned over the toilet seat, and let the mother sit and relax so that her bottom parts are submerged in the healing liquid. Carefully pat dry afterward and pour the used tea into the toilet. This should be repeated several times daily.

To combine these two methods: Use the sitz-bath method, dry off, and allow the bottom tissues to be exposed to fresh clean air (no pants!) for a short while, and then apply the oil and cover up with light cotton underpants with an absorbent, all-natural pad. Repeat this process throughout the two to three days post-partum to ensure speedy healing of tissues and avoid infection.

# Breastfeeding

Generally, breastfeeding does not bring with it any particular diseases or hardships, with most women concerned about only a small handful of issues: producing an acceptable quantity of milk (and drying up the milk when ready), and avoiding or healing mastitis or infections and inflammation in the breast.

## *Producing and Drying Milk*

Herbs that stimulate breast milk production are called galactagogues, and they are generally essential-oil rich and carminative herbs, as well. Their actions stimulate the mammary glands by acting upon the pituitary, particularly through the actions of the chemical compound anethole, which is present in many of the licorice-scented breastfeeding herbs.

The most reliable galactagogues can be taken as teas, candy, tinctures, and capsules, and they are generally made in combinations for flavor and strength. Traditionally, blessed thistle, anise, caraway, dill, fennel seed, mallow, and barley have been used to reliably increase milk production and promote prolactin production. These aromatic herbs are also those very herbs used throughout European history to treat digestive complaints and ease flatulence, making them perform double duty for mothers of infants suffering colic and gas.

To dry up the milk when weaning the baby, mothers turn to astringent herbs. Whereas galactagogues promote prolactin, astringent herbs inhibit prolactin, constrict the mammary ducts, and reduce milk flow and production. Common astringent herbs used for this purpose include sage, yarrow, goldenseal (on the United Plant Savers at-risk list), and to a lesser extent, raspberry. These can be applied topically but are most effective as internal infusions, tinctures, foods, and capsules. Avoid the temptation to squeeze out the milk that is still being produced, as this can stimulate even more production.

## Mastitis

Infection in the mammary glands and milk ducts at any point during breastfeeding is, unfortunately, common and painful. Milk ducts may become clogged, resulting in pain, inflammation, redness, and a hard swelling on the infected breast, and infection may set in, which can cause fever. The causes of mastitis are many: compression of the breast (sleeping positions, etc.), cracked nipples leading to infection by *Staphylococcus, Streptococcus,* or *E. coli* pathogens,[73] use of a breast pump, and even diabetes or steroid use. Mastitis makes breastfeeding uncomfortable and painful, but more breastfeeding is often exactly the remedy that helps the most. The more frequently a baby nurses, the more likely a plugged duct is to clear.

Anti-inflammatory and antimicrobial herbs are the best choices to directly treat a case of mastitis; there are many folk remedies, indicating this age-old condition was well recognized historically. The topical application of warm cabbage was a common treatment, likely since cabbage was common and because it has the ability to, like plantain, absorb heat from the body.

### Herbal Anti-Inflammatories for Topical Use in Mastitis

| | | |
|---|---|---|
| plantain | yarrow | violet |
| arnica | white willow | vervain |
| turmeric | ginger | cabbage |

*Internal* anti-inflammatories acceptable during breastfeeding include vervain, valerian, cramp bark, and ginger. Treat concurrent symptoms such as fever, aches, and fatigue with the appropriate herbs (mentioned elsewhere in this book).

---

73   Romm (2010), 450.

Reducing stress to allow for proper let-down of milk is also key. Stress can interfere with the natural hormonal drive to produce breast milk, so anxiolytic herbs and nervine tonics can be very beneficial for the mother whose milk supply won't start or has diminished. Specific stress relieving herbs appropriate for breastfeeding include skullcap, hops, lemon balm, lavender, motherwort, vervain, chamomile, and oats milky tops. Provide the mother quiet time when she is free from displaying the new baby to relatives; she needs alone time and time with her baby free from distractions, socializing, and the expectations of hosting well-wishers.

For a discussion of post-partum depression and mother's stress, see chapter 6.

Long the territory of midwives, herbal support for the pregnant and nursing mother is being shared with the wider healing community in an effort to make these remedies known and to offer as many options and choices as possible to the mother. Her informed decisions can only be made when she has the support from her caregivers as well as the legal right to choose her own methods of nourishment and treatment, for both herself and her baby. Using herbs during pregnancy, childbirth, lactation, and weaning is a safe and honorable way to support families during these meaningful experiences.

# CHAPTER FOURTEEN

# Menopause

Historically, aging women were viewed in two very opposing ways: ma-triarchal and women-centered societies viewed aging women as the wise crone, appreciating her wisdom and valuing her opinions. She was a leader and involved in family matters, politics, local government, business, reli-gious leadership, and education. Many cultures demonstrated this type of positive treatment for their elder women: Native American nations, Ca-naanites, Egyptians, and ancient Babylonians and Sumerians. But when men-centered societies and patriarchies invaded these civilizations, espe-cially after the appearance of the Proto-Indo-Europeans,[74] they stamped out this veneration of the woman (of any age) and paved the way for later societies, such as medieval Europe's, to view elder and aging women not only as useless but actually as evil. Old women were portrayed not as wise

---

74   Stone (1976).

and helpful but as hysterical and even as witches. The massacre of millions throughout the centuries of the witch craze was not a sudden accident but the culmination of centuries of misogyny and hatred toward women.

Thankfully, our culture and others are beginning to understand the misery of this type of thinking. American women's suffrage (right to vote) in 1920 and the Feminist Movement of the 1960s and 70s brought attention to the fact that there has been a great disparity between the sexes for far too long. This type of inequality affects not only payroll and job opportunities, but also women's health during natural cycles such as ovulation, menstruation, and menopause.

It is helpful to understand just how cyclical women are. There are many ancient myths that celebrate the cycles of which women form an integral part: the story of the Greek goddess Demeter mirrors women's cycles of flowing and drying. Cultures all over the world celebrate the connection between women and the moon (*moon, mind, menstrual,* and *menopause* share the same Proto-Indo European etymology). Many goddesses are associated with the moon, including the Greek Artemis, Hawaiian Hina, Babylonian Ishtar, Korean Dae-Soon, Roman Diana, Greek (and possibly older) Hecate, Roman Luna, and Chinese Kwan Yin, to name a few. While societies have abused women's relationship to the moon's cycles, using moon-related terms such as *lunatic* against women, women can pull strength from the symbolism implied in the always waning/always waxing moon to support their experience of menopause.

## What Is Menopause?

Menopause is the physiological experience of the cessation of the menstrual cycle. Specifically, perimenopause is the time leading up to menopause, with women experiencing decreased estrogen, decreased progesterone, fewer eggs produced, less endometrium, shorter and more erratic cycles, and the end of ovulation. Menopause is considered complete after twelve months have passed without ovulation. The woman's reproductive experience begins with menarche, extends through fertility for twenty to forty years, enters the climacteric (including perimenopause), and finally the reproductive experience ends with menopause.

Hormones are at the center of each of these stages. Throughout a woman's normal menstrual cycle, estrogen is produced in a number of locations in the body such as the ovaries and the adrenal glands, and it's converted from some foods. Progesterone is only produced after ovulation, and it comes from the ovaries and the adrenal glands. After menopause, the adrenal glands take over full production of estrogen until about age seventy.

Because of the spike in estrogen at ovulation and then the lesser spike of progesterone after ovulation, we know that estrogen is generally produced in higher amounts than progesterone. But the balance between the two is essential to avoid emotional and physical problems. Too much estrogen and too little progesterone can trigger a painful imbalance. Excess estrogen can cause bloating, fatigue, weight gain, blood clots, breast tenderness, and other PMS symptoms that can reappear during perimenopause. Hormone replacement therapy and estrogen replacement therapy generally replace only estrogen, ignoring progesterone, which can lead to greater imbalance.

Progesterone is a very vital hormone that needs to appear, even in minimal doses, until menopause is complete. Progesterone does the following:

- Helps burn fat for energy

- Decreases water retention

- Decreases hot flashes

- Attaches to GABA receptor in the brain to ease depression, mood swings, and anxiety

- Improves mental function and clarity by protecting the myelin sheath around nerve cells

- Improves relaxation for good sleep and eases insomnia

- Increases the sex drive

- Balances thyroid function (to avoid weight gain, fatigue, food cravings and low blood sugar)

Progesterone also increases the efficacy of other hormones like thyroid stimulating hormone, testosterone, and estrogen. The following herbs can be used to increase estrogen and/or progesterone levels:

### Estrogenic (Estrogen-Increasing) Herbs

- **angelica** (*Angelica archangelica; A. sinensis*): also called dong quai, this herb does not possess phytoestrogens (that we know of) but instead contains coumarins; this may explain its emmenagogic action (stimulating the uterus) and why angelica is contraindicated with certain drugs, including warfarin. Dong quai is a traditional tier 1 tonic for menopause and can be a tier 2 specific for nervousness, insomnia, hot flashes, and mental fog.

- **hops** (*Humulus lupulus*): may present estrogenic actions especially relevant in hot flashes leading to insomnia.

- **sage** (*Salvia* spp.): may present estrogenic actions especially relevant in hot flashes, excessive sweating, heart palpitations, and panic.

- **red clover** (*Trifolium pratense*): has estrogenic effects on endometrial and breast cancer cells in vitro. Contains isoflavones similar to soy.

- **black cohosh** (*Actaea racemosa*): this North American native wildflower has long been used, and is widely currently used, for menopausal symptoms, including hot flashes, menstrual disorders including amenorrhea, and PMS. It is not clear whether black cohosh has an actual estrogen effect in the body or whether it mimics estrogen or works in an altogether different manner.

- **soy** (*Glycine max*): the high-protein soybean is a source of phytoestrogens in the form of isoflavones and are believed to be partly responsible for milder symptoms in people whose diets include soy.

- **flax** (*Linum* spp.): high in lignans (phytoestrogens). Easy to include in the diet, flax reduces total and LDL cholesterol.

- **licorice** (*Glycyrrhiza glabra*): an excellent adrenal support herb, licorice is soothing and anti-inflammatory and makes a good tier 3 corollary herb during menopause, but because it can cause water retention and high blood pressure, it should not be used long-term nor by those with hypertension.

### Possible Progesterone (Progesterone-Increasing) Herbs

The following herbs have traditionally been used to support progesterone-like effects in the body although neither directly increases progesterone. Further study and work with a phytotheraphy professional is needed.

- **wild yam** (*Dioscorea villosa*): contains the sterol saponin, which resembles progesterone but cannot be converted naturally by the body into progesterone. Unclear whether internal natural wild yam herbal remedies can increase progesterone in the body; its action may lie in its influence on other endocrine organs or systems.

- **chaste tree berry** (*Vitex agnus-castus*): widely labeled a hormone regulator, likely because it "balances" the pituitary and particularly the HPA axis. Can be taken long-term for anxiety associated with PMS or menopause, but is contraindicated in pregnancy.

Soy also contains the saponins that resemble progesterone, though soy is most commonly used to increase estrogen.

Many women find body temperature to be greatly affected during peri-menopause and menopause. Herbs with symptomatic relief as warming or cooling agents include:

| Warming Herbs | Warming Herbs | Cooling Herbs | Cooling Herbs |
|---|---|---|---|
| wild sarsaparilla | ginseng | mallow | chickweed |
| smilax | sassafras | licorice | spearmint |
| helonias | angelica | chamomile | violet |
| sage | yarrow | ashwagandha | rose |
| cinnamon | rhodiola | elder flower | linden |
| ginger | peppermint | lemon balm | oats milky tops |

## Menopause Formulas
### A Formula for Hot Flashes

> › 1 part black cohosh
>
> › 1 part wild sarsaparilla
>
> › 1 part hops
>
> › 1 part ginseng

### A Formula for Emotional Swings

> › 2 parts vervain
>
> › 1 part wild yam
>
> › 1 part chaste tree berry
>
> › 1 part St. John's wort
>
> › 1 part lemon balm

## Adrenal Nourishment During Menopause

When the endocrine system registers an emergency or a stressful situation, it responds with the self-protective symptoms including increased heartbeat, pupil dilation, redirection of blood and energy from the periphery to the heart, rapid breathing, and muscle contractions; afterward, the person experiences fatigue and confusion. Some of these same symptoms are observed in the normal menopausal woman, and we can recognize some of the stress of hormone changes affecting the adrenal glands with "life threatening" urgency.

The hormone-secreting adrenals are already under excessive stress since the ovaries have ceased producing their fair share of estrogen and progesterone. Add to this the normal stress associated with being a mother, grandmother, executive, politician and/or professional, and you have a woman whose endocrine system is reacting to stress.

Typical perimenopause symptoms such as hot flashes, rapid heart beat, vaginal dryness, sweating, rapid breathing, muscle aches, confusion or mental fog, and fatigue can often be explained by adrenal stress. It makes sense to approach issues of perimenopause as if you were addressing adrenal insufficiency—with adrenal supportive and adaptogenic herbs that nourish and tone the endocrine system. I've had excellent results working with menopausal women by supporting their adrenal health using lemon balm and licorice, among other herbs; they report their feelings of anxiety, scattered thinking, and physical symptoms have diminished.

### Adrenal Nourishers

In addition to licorice, vervain, and black cohosh, consider:

- **eleuthero** (*Eleutherococcus senticosus*): also called Siberian ginseng, this herb is generally used for stamina and endurance and to support the immune system. It is an effective choice for menopausal women undergoing an extreme transition and feel exhausted or depleted, or who are at risk for contracting viral or bacterial infections. Can be used as a tier 1 tonic or tier 2 specific.

- **lemon balm** (*Melissa officinalis*): effective for focus, feelings of confidence and satisfaction; specific against restlessness and panic. Antiviral. Can be taken long-term.

## Nervine Tonics

In addition to chamomile, passionflower, skullcap and lemon balm, consider:

- **oats** (*Avena sativa*): excellent long-term tier 1 tonic for the menopausal woman, especially in cases of frazzled nerves, exhaustion, or weepy emotions. Also applicable in cases of anger and excessive heat. Combines well with lavender and nettle.
- **motherwort** (*Leonurus cardiaca*): tier 1 tonic or tier 2 specific for the menopausal woman who feels panic or fear, or whose restlessness causes heart tremors or other cardiac stress. Also, as a bitter, for the woman whose digestion has shifted or changed as a result of hormone imbalance.

## Sedatives

In addition to chamomile (a mild bitter), consider valerian and hops for the menopausal woman experiencing insomnia especially due to night hot flashes or anger. Consider rose, ashwagandha, lavender, and oats for the woman who cannot sleep due to incessant thinking and "brain overdrive."

## Hepatic Herbs

Support the liver's work at excreting metabolic waste properly. As the body's production of hormones declines, spent and extra hormones must be removed from the bloodstream effectively. While yarrow is a hepatic herb, it tends to be warming, which most menopausal women don't need. Instead, consider cooling or neutral hepatics such as motherwort, burdock root, dandelion root, and milk thistle.

*Adrenal Nourishment Formulas*

### A FORMULA FOR PERIMENOPAUSE WITH INSOMNIA

- › 2 parts skullcap
- › 1 part nettle
- › 1 part passionflower
- › 1 part hops

### A FORMULA FOR PERIMENOPAUSE WITH HEADACHES AND DRYNESS

- › 2 parts ginkgo
- › 1 part mullein
- › 1 part feverfew
- › 1 part black cohosh

### A FORMULA FOR PERIMENOPAUSE WITH ANXIETY

- › 2 parts vervain
- › 2 parts motherwort
- › 1 part nettle
- › 1 part ashwagandha

### A FORMULA FOR POST-MENOPAUSE WITH HEART PALPITATIONS

- › 2 parts motherwort
- › 1 part ginkgo
- › 1 part hawthorn
- › 1 part linden

# CHAPTER FIFTEEN

# The Endocrine System

The endocrine system is composed of glands that secrete hormones that influence a wide range of bodily functions, including physical functions such as weight loss, weight gain, digestive function, and temperature regulation, as well as emotional functions such as moods. A highly complex system of this-triggers-that, the endocrine system is a maturing branch of science that is an excellent example of how herbal remedies are not necessarily "organ" specific but, rather, are used based on their action, which can affect an organ, an entire system, or a complex interplay between systems. In other words, there is seldom one particular herb that "cures" one particular organ, especially with endocrine glands; rather, a broad range of herbs may exert many diverse actions upon a gland and its connected systems that brings about a desired response.

The endocrine system is complex and expansive, but here we will focus on some of the most common illnesses and conditions arising from an imbalance of glandular function. In particular, we will discuss the interplay between the hypothalamus, the pituitary, the thyroid, and the adrenals. These form various "axis" through which the hormones are expressed. The hypothalamus sends messages to, among other glands, the pituitary, which is in the forefront of the brain. From here, the pituitary sends signals to many organs and glands including the ovaries and gonads, and for our purposes here, especially to the adrenals and the thyroid, forming the hypothalamic pituitary adrenal (HPA) axis and the hypothalamic pituitary thyroid (HPT) axis. A truly in-depth analysis of this system is beyond the scope of this book, but here we will cover the basic information required to make educated decisions about herbal remedies that may or may not influence dysfunctions of the thyroid and the adrenals.

First: the **hypothalamus**. Located just below the thalamus above the brain stem, in roughly the central part of the brain, the hypothalamus controls metabolic function and serves as a "link" between the endocrine system and the nervous system. The hypothalamus receives input from the central nervous system, sensory organs such as the nose, and the cerebral cortex; from these "directions" this tiny organ controls the pituitary gland by releasing thyrotropin and other hormones. The hypothalamus is the origin, the first stimulus, for many of the hormones and pre-hormones released by the pituitary and other glands, but it also directly releases some hormones of its own, including gonadotropin-releasing hormone, dopamine, and oxytocin (which stimulates uterine contraction and lactation for new mothers). Generally, however, herbal treatment for issues relating to metabolism or glandular function isn't directed at the hypothalamus but rather at the gland in question.

Second: the **pituitary**. The hypothalamus stimulates its close neighbor the pituitary to secrete a number of hormones that will affect the thyroid and the adrenals, among others. Specifically, the combined anterior and posterior pituitary, which is a small gland that rests just below the hypothalamus and adjacent to the optic nerve, secretes nine hormones, including:

- Follicle-stimulating hormone (FSH), which stimulates the maturation of the ovarian follicles (egg) in the ovary in women and the creation of sperm in men
- Luteinizing hormone (LH) which stimulates ovulation, among other actions
- Prolactin, which stimulates milk production for nursing mothers
- Oxytocin, which regulates contractions during labor

From the pituitary, two other primary glands are put to work: the thyroid and the adrenals.

## Hypothalamic Pituitary Adrenal (HPA) Axis

The adrenal glands, which sit atop the kidneys, are comprised of the adrenal cortex and the adrenal medulla, each of which secretes specialized hormones that:

- Stimulate inflammatory response
- Regulate metabolism
- Manage reactionary response (the fight-or-flight response)
- Engage pupil dilation
- Suppress or stimulate the immune system
- And even direct complex intra-endocrine systems such as sodium reabsorption by the kidneys

The adrenals are generally credited with our "stress" response (though this response originates in the hypothalamus), as these glands produce adrenaline (epinephrine) and noradrenaline (norepinephrine) that ready the brain and the body's muscles for sudden action by boosting their supply of oxygen and sugars, increasing the heart rate, and stimulating vasodilation. The adrenal medulla even secretes dopamine that increases heart rate and blood pressure, and enkaphalin, which regulates and often mitigates the brain's perception of pain—essential in acute stress situations.

Herbal actions usually required to assist and support the adrenals include herbs that normalize an acute response to stress, that soothe the central nervous system, and that bring normalcy back to the digestive and cardiovascular systems: adaptogens, anxiolytics, nervine tonics, amphoterics, mild-to-moderate sedatives, and bitters. Since there is no magic "adrenal herb," herbalists employ a wide range of herbs with the required actions to generally assist and support the entire endocrine-nervous system relationship, focusing on nervine tonics that allow the body to better adapt to stress. In addition, hepatic and alterative herbs are used in many adrenal formulas because: (1) stressful situations may cause changes in the hypothalamus that adversely affect the amounts and kinds of hormones subsequently released from the pituitary and other glands on the axis, (2) excessive hormones circulating in the bloodstream can adversely affect the natural balance and feedback mechanisms to the hypothalamus, and (3) environmental toxins can also play a role in disrupting the endocrine process.

The following lists indicate the most common herbs used for the desired herbal action to influence the glands of the endocrine system.

## Nervous System Herbs for Adrenal Support

| NERVINE TONICS (MILDEST) | ANXIOLYTICS (MODERATE) | ADAPTOGENS (STRONGEST) |
|---|---|---|
| lemon balm | ashwagandha | rhodiola |
| oats milky tops | skullcap | licorice |
| motherwort | St. John's wort | ginseng |
| vervain | passionflower | eleuthero |

| Nervine Tonics (mildest) | Anxiolytics (moderate) | Adaptogens (strongest) |
|---|---|---|
| valerian | | schisandra |
| chamomile | | holy basil |
| rose | | |
| nettles | | |

### *Adrenal Gland Formulas*
#### A Formula for Adrenal Support
> › 2 parts oats milky tops
>
> › 1 part motherwort
>
> › 1 part eleuthero
>
> › 1 part chamomile

A note about **lavender:** lavender is often grouped under sedative and even nervine herbs, but it can have a very intense effect, especially on children and sensitive people. To some, lavender can be not only stimulating but also be irritating and can cause headaches, muscle tension, and more. For these reasons, I do not list lavender as an adrenal tier 1 tonic.

## Hypothalamus Pituitary Thyroid Axis

As with the HPA Axis, all activity begins in the hypothalamus, goes through the pituitary, but then redirects to the thyroid when the pituitary produces thyroid stimulating hormones, or TSH. This hormone, in turn, stimulates the secretion of thyroxine, a hormone involved in the regulation of the heart rate, digestive activity, body temperature (especially through sweating), and even calorie consumption: in other words, metabolism. Typical disorders include hypothyroidism (low thyroid function), hyperthyroidism (excessive thyroid function), and nodules or cancers.

An enlarged thyroid is called goiter, which displays as a large swollen mass on the neck.

## Hypothyroidism

Hypothyroidism is low thyroid hormone, or underactivity of the thyroid. Hypothyroidism can be caused by too little stimulus from the pituitary as well as problems within the thyroid itself. Symptoms of poor thyroid function include weight gain (despite loss of appetite), fatigue, hair loss, bradycardia (insufficient heart rate that minimizes oxygen availability to organs), goiter, and inability to properly regulate body temperature, resulting in constant "cold." Hypothyroidism can be a genetic predisposition, or it can be brought on by other illnesses (such as autoimmune disorders or thyroid cancer), or the insufficient absorption of the mineral iodine. Pregnant women with nutrient-deficient diets can give birth to infants with congenital hypothyroidism; many developing countries now routinely screen for hypothyroidism in newborns and administer levothyroxine (a synthetic form of thyroxine) to reverse this common disorder.

Traditional herbal remedies have tended to focus on bladderwrack and kelp, two seaweeds high in iodine and other trace minerals. This therapy can be useful for iodine-deficient hypothyroidism, but only minimally effective for genetically-based illnesses. Other herbal actions are needed to address corollary issues and symptoms that result from low thyroid levels. These include:

- **digestive/carminative:** the digestive system suffers as a result of poor thyroid function; warming and aromatic carminative herbs can stimulate sluggish digestion and stimulate the body to secrete natural digestive enzymes to improve the overall digestive process. Better digestion can lead to better absorption of necessary trace minerals.

- **warming/stimulating:** warm cooked foods and warming herbs can stimulate the circulatory system, the digestion, and even mental processes. Hot mint tea, ginger, cardamom, clove, rosemary, cinnamon, oregano, mustard, and cayenne can all be used as warming stimulating herbs in the diet and as remedies. Many of these can also be made as compresses to alleviate cool congested spots (such as over the abdomen).

- **hepatic:** since the liver metabolizes all bodily hormones, and it flushes spent hormones and toxins from the bloodstream, supporting the liver with hepatic herbs is important in both hypo- and hyperthyroidism. Since dandelion and yellow dock are cooling herbs, milk thistle is a neutral choice for hypothyroid liver care.

- **antidepressant:** the body and mind are naturally sedated and "down" in hypothyroidism, so it's essential to nourish and revitalize the central nervous system. Rhodiola, ginger, and verbena (drunk as a hot tea) are good tier 2 Specifics and tier 3 corollary herbs.

- **cardiotonics** and **vasoconstrictors:** working with the presumption that cardiovascular tonics and especially vasoconstrictors assist the heart and vesicular systems by way of toning and tightening, thereby stimulating proper circulatory function, herbs that perform this action will be welcome in formulas for people with sluggish systems, poor circulation, cold hands and feet, and slow metabolism. Use gentle cardiotonics and gentle vasoconstrictors such as prickly ash, as the intent is to support and tone, not to overly stimulate. Work with the person's primary care provider to ensure proper balance for the cardiovascular system.

- **adaptogen:** herbs such as eleuthero can provide a mild adaptive action for those who need a physical and mental "boost" that is long-term and sustained;

- **tonic:** though many tonics are sedative (or at least calming), tonics for the hypothyroid person need to be warming, nutritive, and uplifting. These can include hot drinks or tinctures of: nettle, hot mint, ginger, hawthorn, rhodiola, and schisandra.

- **thyroid stimulating:** few herbs seem to directly stimulate the thyroid safely. While bladderwrack affects the gland, researchers are unclear how it works and how it raises or lowers iodine levels.

### *Hypothyroid Formulas*
#### A FORMULA FOR HYPOTHYROIDISM DUE TO INSUFFICIENT IODINE

> 2 parts eleuthero

> 1 part bladderwrack

> 1 part ginger

> 1 part cleavers

#### A FORMULA FOR GENETIC HYPOTHYROIDISM

> 2 parts schisandra

> 1 part eleuthero

> 1 part milk thistle

> 1 part motherwort

### *Hyperthyroidism*

Hyperthyroidism is excessive thyroid function, where the thyroid hormones over-produce. This process can cause goiter (as can hypothyroidism) as well as the physical and emotional symptoms that arise from hyperthyroid production. Graves' disease is the most common culprit behind hyperthyroidism, and it is primarily genetic with a high proportion of sufferers being women. Many cases are diagnosed in teenagers, with some cases occurring post-partum. Symptoms of hyperthyroidism include excessive sweating, weight loss despite an increased appetite, muscle weakness, and heart palpitations; symptoms of Graves' disease include hyperthyroid symptoms plus more extreme hypertension, excessive sweating and inability to tolerate heat, hyperactivity, opthalmopathy, irritability and depression. The body's metabolism is in overdrive, with digestion, cardiac, and body temperature regulation amped up and uncontrolled.

Tier 2 Specifics for hyperthyroidism include:

- **lemon balm** (*Melissa officinalis*): normalizes an overactive thyroid. Lemon balm has been shown in *in-vitro* studies to block thyroid stimulating hormone receptors, inhibiting the binding of bovine TSH to human thyroid tissues, and also inhibiting the binding of autoantibodies in Graves' disease. Best taken as a cool tea, syrup, capsule, or tincture.

- **motherwort** (*Leonurus cardiaca*): motherwort addresses heart arrhythmia, tachycardia (excessive heart rate), and palpitations—in addition to being the go-to herb for women with anxiety and nervous tension, it is a specific for both hypertension and hyperthyroidism. Bitter motherwort is best taken as a capsule or tincture.

For hypertension, cardiac tonic herbs are invaluable—really the core of the therapy, tier 2 Specifics. Consider hawthorn, bugleweed, ginkgo, linden, and motherwort.

Additional actions for hyperthyroidism are cooling, calming, tonic, and digestive:

- **carminatives:** since people with hyperthyroidism suffer with increased body heat, cooling and aromatic herbs are needed. Cooling tier 1 tonic or tier 3 corollary herbs include spearmint, chamomile, lemon balm, dill, fennel, catnip, burdock, chickweed, elderflower, red clover, and lavender.
- **respiratory tonics:** gentle support includes mullein, elderflower, and elderberry.
- **immune support:** hyperthyroid conditions, particularly Graves' disease, can impair the immune system—however since Graves' creates an autoimmune condition, immune support must be very nourishment-based rather than immunostimulatory. Many immune support herbs are rather too strong, hot, and stimulating for use in hyperthyroid conditions, so seek out the cooler, calming immune-supportive herbs: elderberry and elderflower are ideal, as are calendula, sage, lemon balm, spilanthes, nettle, self-heal, astragalus, rose hips, and a variety of medicinal mushrooms including maitake, reishi, agaricus, and shiitake.
- **antioxidant:** consider decaffeinated green tea, bilberries, blueberries.

## *Hyperthyroid Formulas*
### A FORMULA FOR HYPERTHYROIDISM
> › 2 parts lemon balm
> › 2 parts chamomile
> › 1 part motherwort
> › 1 part hawthorn

### A Formula for Hyperthyroidism with Frequent Viral Sickness

› 2 parts lemon balm

› 1 part elderflower

› 1 part motherwort

› 1 part St. John's wort

### A Formula for Hyperthyroidism with Heart Palpitations

› 2 parts motherwort

› 1 part hawthorn

› 1 part linden

› 1 part rose

As always, work in partnership with the client's support team and with other healing arts practitioners, and use herbs and herbal remedies as a foundation for supporting endocrine health.

# CHAPTER SIXTEEN

# Herbal Healing for Men

Lest men begin to feel their needs cannot be met by plants because of all the attention given to women's body systems, men are just as connected to plants and receptive to their actions and guidance as women. Men's bodies respond just as well to plants as women's bodies though their needs for the actions of plants differ in significant ways. Men's needs for the spiritual connection with nature is also strong, vibrant, and centered on a compassionate reawakening that can be explored through the ancient myths and herbal heritage of many cultures.

While both men and women experience similar digestive upset, respiratory and cardiovascular risks described in the previous chapters, men's reproductive systems differ broadly from women's. Plant medicines have been used for centuries to address issues specific to men's reproduction and to nourish and support men's continued health.

## Prostate Problems

Nearly half of all men over age forty-five suffer some sort of prostate problem, whether mild or benign inflammation; benign prostatic hypertrophy (BPH); or prostate cancer, a leading cause of death among men. Herbs have a rightful place in prostate therapies for both nutritive and supportive functions. Benign prostatic hypertrophy or prostatic enlargement can restrict fluid flow from the kidneys to the bladder, resulting in infection. Anti-inflammatory and antimicrobial herbs are key in these cases, as are diuretic and demulcent herbs. The following herbs can be used in almost any tier of the 4-tier formula:

- **saw palmetto** (*Serenoa repens*): this palm tree native to the southeastern United States was historically used by the Seminole nation for basketry, fans, rope, tools, cordage, and other household materials; the berries were eaten for food. Used for the male genitourinary system especially for urinary incontinence (often a symptom of prostate problems) and for weakened reproductive organs in both sexes. [75] Its use for treating prostate cancer is inconsistent with its eclectic use of remediating urinary dysfunction, but because of the proximity of the prostate gland and the gland's literal "wrapping" around the urethra, the use of saw palmetto in recent years has focused on treating prostate cancer. The berries are tinctured or dried and encapsulated as a remedy specific to the prostate gland; though clinical trials are mixed in their results[76], saw palmetto shows some improvement in nocturia and other symptoms of BPH. Extracts of the berry appear to be antiandrogenic and both antiestrogenic and estrogenic. [77]

---

75  Hoffmann (1996).

76  Thompson Healthcare Inc. (2007).

77  Ibid.

Time will tell if this herb truly does impact human hormones or resist the growth of prostate cancer cells. Until these findings are made, it is safe to use saw palmetto to treat urinary symptoms (associated with BPH and otherwise) and as a male reproductive and urinary tonic.

- **nettle** (*Urtica dioica*): while nettle leaves feature in herbal heritage for other issues, it is the root we turn to now. The radix of the nettle plant has come to light fairly recently as a key prostate remedy though its mechanism of action is unclear. It appears to have anti-inflammatory properties that make it useful alongside saw palmetto. Its folk history suggests marked improvement in urinary flow and urinary tract strength, especially in the presence of an enlarged prostate gland, without necessarily acting upon the size of the prostate gland directly.

- **pygeum** (*Prunus africana*): this relative of the cherry tree has been the subject of clinical and scientific studies; it is anti-inflammatory specific to the genitourinary tract, and it is seen to improve bladder function. [78]

- **yarrow** (*Achillea millefolium*): both diuretic and antimicrobial, yarrow serves as a tier 4 vehicle herb and can be a tier 3 corollary herb for the urinary system and prostate.

- **ginger** (*Zingiber officinale*): warming, antimicrobial, vasodilatory, carminative, and diuretic, ginger can be a key tier 3 or tier 4 in prostate formulas.

- **turmeric** (*Curcuma longa*): highly regarded as an anti-inflammatory, especially for the integumentary system, turmeric can be useful in cases of prostate inflammation where cramping, swelling, and inflammation are prominent symptoms.

---

78   Ibid.

- **mallow** (*Althea* spp.): this mucilaginous root's cooling (demulcent) and moisturizing properties both internally and externally relieve redness, swelling, heat, and inflammation. Useful post-surgery as well as for general daily support of an inflamed prostate.

- **green tea** (*Camellia sinensis*): antioxidant and diuretic. Caution: contains caffeine.

### *Prostate Formulas*
#### A FORMULA FOR URINARY INCONTINENCE ASSOCIATED WITH BPH

> › 2 parts green tea
>
> › 1 part yarrow
>
> › 1 part pygeum
>
> › 1 part nettle root

#### A FORMULA FOR URINARY BURNING ASSOCIATED WITH BPH

> › 2 parts marshmallow
>
> › 1 part cornsilk
>
> › 1 part saw palmetto
>
> › 1 part yarrow

## Erectile Dysfunction

Erectile dysfunction, or ED, is the physical inability to produce or maintain an erection for sexual purposes. Common underlying causes of ED include stress and anxiety, diabetes (nearly half of all men with diabetes experience ED), hypertension and atherosclerosis, and certain medications for blood pressure or depression that seriously impact erectile function. Additionally, obesity lowers testosterone levels and can lead to lower sex drive and impeded sexual function.

Because of the seriousness of the underlying causes (that may be unknown to the man experiencing ED) it is important to rule out heart disease, diabetes, or atherosclerosis. Both ED and many potential underlying causes can successfully be treated with herbal medicine. Long-term foundational support using tonics is the best approach while short-term remedies can include caffeine-free stimulants and warming vasodilators. Herbal actions useful for ED include:

- **anti-inflammatories:** saw palmetto, Jamaican dogwood, St. John's wort, plantain, turmeric, ginger.

- **cardiotonics:** hawthorn, garlic, motherwort.

- **vasodilators:** peppermint, ginger, gotu kola. In particular, ginger combined with the stimulants listed below can be taken on an as-needed basis as a hot tea or cordial.

- **nervine tonics:** oatstraw and oats milky tops, lemon balm, motherwort, passionflower, St. John's wort.

- **adaptogens:** eleuthero, *panax ginseng*, echinacea.

- **stimulants:** not referring to stimulants such as caffeine or nootropic drugs, but rather herbs that uplift and warm the body, such as wild sarsaparilla, ginger, peppermint, cayenne, all bitters.

## Erectile Dysfunction Formulas
### A Formula for Erectile Dysfunction

> › 2 parts hawthorn
> › 1 part peppermint
> › 1 part saw palmetto
> › 1 part ginger

## Another Formula for Erectile Dysfunction

› 2 parts eleuthero

› 1 part wild sarsaparilla

› 1 part Jamaican dogwood

› 1 part garlic

# Energy

A brief discussion of yang and yin will be useful here: in Traditional Chinese Medicine and Taoist teachings, the dualities or complementary opposing energies of male and female extend to medicine and to the functions of the human body as well as plants. This fascinating understanding of opposites and energetic forces can be applied to all of life (and death) and is exhibited throughout the day (and night) by the beauty (and brutality) of everything. In mythology, many cultures associate the cool, dark, moonlit night with female energies and the hot, bright sun-filled day with male energies. Of course, all people and all herbs exhibit and experience some of each, and the balance can be appreciated in healthy, robust, compassionate men and women. But for the purposes of healing illnesses with plant medicines, it is useful to recognize some of these qualities in plants and associate them with the remediating actions needed.

It would be easy to get carried away by the complex poetry of the yin-yang philosophy, but its essence (and its application in herbal formulary) is this:

| Yang | Yang | Yin | Yin |
|---|---|---|---|
| Energy | Herbal Action | Energy | Herbal Action |
| male | | female | |
| hot | warming | cool | emollient |

| YANG | YANG | YIN | YIN |
|---|---|---|---|
| dry | astringent | wet | demulcent |
| fast | vasodilating | slow | vasoconstricting |
| light | | dark | cooling |
| hard | vulnerary | soft | moisturizing |
| aggressive | rubefacient | yielding | tonic |
| stimulating | stimulant | passive | nutritive |
| | carminative | soothing/relaxing | sedative |

For men lacking in stamina, enduring a cold, congested, or weakening illness, passing through a stressful time that leads to depression, confusion, or a desire to do nothing, yang herbs may assist both emotionally and physically. Herbs that promote healthy, sustained, and usually yang energy include:

- yarrow
- ginger
- cayenne pepper
- garlic
- wild sarsaparilla
- ginseng
- peppermint
- black tea
- damiana

These herbs are used on an as-needed basis and are not tonics in Western herbal medicine. Ayurvedic medicine, however, considers bitters and stimulants good tonics for recuperating, to be used for the duration of convalescence in conjunction with yin herbs and foods for cooling, soothing, and nourishing.

# Stress

As mentioned previously, stress can be addressed using nervine tonics and adaptogens. In my experience, I've found that men tend to benefit from ginseng more than women, for whom this adaptogenic herb can be too stimulating and have a "caffeine-like" effect, sometimes causing gastric irritation. Men also benefit from the calming, steadying effects of herbs such as spearmint, oats, and lemon balm, as well as the more "yang" effects of herbs such as yarrow, peppermint, and wild sarsaparilla. See chapter 6 for more details about nervous system and tonic herbs. Also see glossary D for discussions about tier 1 tonic herbs.

## *Stress Formulas*
### A FORMULA FOR MEN'S CHRONIC STRESS

> › 2 parts oats milky tops

> › 1 part schisandra

> › 1 part ginger

> › 1 part lemon balm

### A FORMULA FOR MEN'S STRESS WITH DEBILITY AND EMOTIONAL FATIGUE

> › 2 parts catnip

> › 1 part eleuthero or ginseng

> › 1 part yarrow

> › 1 part peppermint

## Hair Loss and Balding

Male pattern and female pattern balding is known as androgenic alopecia, and is a very common presentation in certain genetic populations where receding and thinning hair develops with age. Male pattern balding can begin as early as age twelve, with most susceptible men experiencing its effects by age fifty. Though there are no direct herbal remedies known to address male or female pattern baldness, certain plants help indirectly; folk plant wisdom points to a few plants that may diminish the effects of this apparently genetic condition. Plants that are nourishing and nutritive, those that are cerebral stimulators and vasodilators, and those that are antimicrobial may help alleviate the worst of male pattern baldness.

- **nourishing:** nettle leaf is among the top micronutrient herbs, and its regular ingestion can help with general health and hair growth.

- **cerebral tonics:** ginkgo, gotu kola, and lemon balm all stimulate the flow of blood to the brain, which may or may not directly affect the growth of hair.

- **vasodilators:** warming ginger, cayenne, and yarrow are considered "male" tonic herbs for various body systems, and their inclusion in a formula may be useful for opening the arteries and veins for better blood flow and higher oxygen content in the bloodstream. Also consider hawthorn.

- **antimicrobial:** because microbial pathogens have been implicated in certain cases of hair loss, rinsing the scalp with a topical wash of antimicrobial rosemary may relieve the scalp of damaging and clogging oils and residues that impede the growth of hair.

Herbal healing for men involves attention to cycles and natural rhythms, interest in mental and emotional health, and formulas that support the physical needs of the adolescent, adult, and aging man. With proper exercise and attention to diet, men's health is successfully supported using botanical remedies.

# CHAPTER SEVENTEEN

# The Urinary System

The human body has a remarkable array of organs devoted to getting rid of waste. Our lungs breathe out toxic carbon dioxide; our sinuses and even our ears evacuate foreign matter; our skin releases toxins through sweat; and our digestive system eliminates unneeded foods.

Elimination of metabolic waste is the responsibility of the excretory system, a system of channels, tubes, and organs that filters toxins and spent materials from the bloodstream and then shunts them out of the orifices of the body without us having to think about them at all. We covered the colon and the liver, two primary organs of elimination (the liver especially for metabolic processes), in chapter 3, Digestion. Here we'll discuss the urinary system, its function and processes, its potential diseases, and herbal treatments.

# Urinary System Function

One of the body's primary wastes is urine, comprised mainly of the nitrogenous substance urea. Urine generally contains water, proteins, salts, spent hormones, and ammonia, which gives its characteristic odor. The expulsion of urine from the urethra and the body (peeing) is known as urination or micturition.

With its primary function of removing urea from the blood, the urinary system is a substantial filter for our body. Urea, which is produced when a person eats proteins, is sent to the kidneys. These little organs rest along the bottom of a person's back (the adrenal glands sit on top of them), and they are comprised of filtering units called nephrons, which are comprised of blood capillaries and tiny tubes called renal tubules. Urea and other waste, in the liquid form of urine, travels through the nephrons and then through the renal tubules. From here, small amounts of urine flow through two narrow eight- to twelve-inch long tubes called ureters, constantly being pushed by muscle contractions downward into the bladder every ten to fifteen seconds. In the bladder, sphincter muscles can keep the urine from leaking through the urethra and to the outside of the body for up to five hours in most people. In men, the prostate gland is located at the base of the bladder and literally wraps around the urethra.

# Problems of the Urinary System

The following issues are commonly associated with urinary malfunction or disease, all of which can be addressed using *materia medica* and, in some cases, additional diagnosis from a health professional.

### Muscle Debility

If the muscles regulating the direction and flow of the urine become lax due to age or injury, then urine can clog or get backed up, leading to infection. Muscle laxness can also cause urinary incontinence, which leads to leaking. Herbal actions needed include nutritive, circulatory tonics, nervine tonics, astringents.

## Infection

All parts of the urinary system can get infected, including the kidneys (renal infection or acute renal/kidney failure), the bladder (painful bladder syndrome or interstitial cystitis), the nephrons (nephritis), and the ureters (urinary tract infection). Herbal actions needed include antimicrobial, diuretic, hepatic, demulcent, antispasmodic.

## Prostate Problems

Benign prostatic hypertrophy or prostatic enlargement can restrict fluid flow from the kidneys to the bladder, resulting in infection. Consider prostate supportive herbs such as saw palmetto, nettle root, green tea, and pygeum as well as antilithics, antispasmodic, anodyne.

## Proteinuria

Excessive protein in the urine indicates the kidneys may not be functioning at peak. Herbal actions may include diuretics, hepatics, nutritives, and cardiotonics.

## Kidney Stones

Calculi are the "stones," "crystals," or "gravel" formed anywhere in the urinary system. The stone consists of proteins and any of a variety of crystals, including calcium, oxalates, phosphate, and carbonates found in herbs and foods, such as oxalic acid in wood sorrel and spinach. Uric acid can also form stones, and many stones pose the risk of blocking the kidney, ureter, or bladder. Indications of calculi include sudden and sharp pain upon urination, fever, sweating, and blood in the urine. Many herbs throughout history have been called "gravel root" or "stone root," referring to their use in removing the mineral build-up of kidney stones; herbs that help reduce the formation or size of kidney stones or calculi, reduce the inflammation, or help expunge the stones from the urinary system are called antilithic and are tier 2 Specifics.

## Symptoms of Urinary Diseases

The following symptoms can occur due to a variety of diseases and need to be evaluated by a health care professional to determine the cause. Herbal remedies can alleviate symptoms and in some cases address underlying causes.

### Dysuria

Painful urination which includes burning, pain, inflammation, and/or spasm. Herbal protocols include demulcents, analgesics, anti-inflammatories, spasmolytics, and anxiolytics.

### Hematuria

Blood in the urine can indicate serious conditions and requires proper diagnosis. Astringents can stop bleeding though may not cure the cause. Antimicrobials can address underlying causes and prevent further infection.

### Edema

Swelling of any part of the body is called edema; swelling associated with congested heart conditions is called dropsy. Urinary incontinence or irregularity can be a symptom along with other more serious symptoms that require medical intervention. Diuretics or astringents can be palliative but they will not address the cause.

Specific tier 2 herbs for many of the above-mentioned issues, organized by action, may include:

## Antilithic

- **Joe Pye weed** (*Eutrochium purpureum*, formerly named *Eupatorium purpureum* or *E. fistulosa*): Joe Pye is a traditional Native American remedy for kidney stones; legend tells us that a Native American healer named Joe Pye traveled up and down the colonies teaching colonists about this herb, who named the plant after him. The root is tinctured.

- **stone root** (*Collinsonia*): a traditional North American remedy for bladder inflammation and kidney stones.

## Antimicrobial

- **yarrow** (*Achillea millefolium*): In urinary distress (of any etiology), tincture or infusion of fresh yarrow can be invaluable. It is strongly antimicrobial, diuretic, and with an "affinity" for the urinary system. Taken hot, it is also diaphoretic.

- **cleavers** (*Galium aparine*): a strong lymph system tonic and "mover" of fluids; appropriate for most urinary tract issues.

- **thyme** (*Thymus vulgaris*) and **oregano** (*Origanum vulgare*): these immune support herbs fight infection both topically and internally.

- **garlic** (*Allium sativum*): taken raw, garlic is a traditional remedy for viral and bacterial infections.

- **bearberry** (*Arcostaphylos uva-ursi*): bear grape is a traditional glycoside-rich ingredient in the smoking mixture kinnickkinnick. It is a specific for conditions of the urinary system as a tincture, capsule, or tea.

- **juniper berries** (*Juniperus communis*): a mild diuretic, supports infection of the bladder or renal system; a strong tier 3 corollary in urinary tract infection.

- **barberry** (*Berberis vulgaris*): Not to be confused with bearberry, *Berberis vulgaris* (European) and *B. canadensis* (American) are antioxidant and historically used to treat infections in the liver and the urinary system. The powerful alkaloid berberine found in the root is a strong antimicrobial. The berries are showing potential as antilithics for breaking up urinary calculi, and for use as a gall bladder tonic.

- **usnea** (*Usnea* spp.): a bitter and astringent lichen, usnea fights urinary tract infections.

## Demulcent

In addition to mallow, plantain, and slippery elm (discussed elsewhere), consider:

- **corn silk** *(Zea mays):* the silky filaments growing at the top of the edible American corn cobs are tinctured or made into infusions to soothe inflamed and infected urethra and for other inflamed urinary issues; demulcent, cooling, diuretic.

- **pipsissewa** (*Chimaphila umbellata*): the leaves of "spotted wintergreen" are used in infusion or tincture to ease and tone the urinary tract, especially during infection. It is a strong diuretic and is listed on the UpS list (see Glossary E).

## Diuretic

Because they "deliver" herbs to the urinary tract, most diuretics are also vehicles and can be used in tier 3 or tier 4 of any urinary formula. In addition to dandelion, yarrow, nettle, stone root, Joe Pye weed, corn silk, bearberry, cleavers, juniper, and pipsissewa, consider:

- **celery seed** (*Apium graveolens*): A traditional remedy for urinary tract disorders, celery seed is a safe and strong diuretic. According to the University of Maryland Medical Center, celery seed is used to increase urine output, help treat arthritis and gout, reduce muscle spasms and inflammation in the urinary tract, and even lower blood pressure.

- **parsley** (*Apium petroselinum*): a close relative of celery, parsley has long been used as a diuretic in Western herbal tradition. The herb is high in vitamins and is a common garnish and culinary herb thanks to its sharp flavor. According to the National Institutes of Health, studies on parsley show that its strong diuretic action is due to its ability to help the body retain potassium. Because the sodium-potassium balance is critical to both nervous system function and cardiovascular function, use caution when placing parsley in any formulas for people with nervous system imbalances, cardiovascular imbalances, high or low blood pressure, or who are pregnant.

## Anti-inflammatory

Consider mallow and licorice, discussed elsewhere. Licorice can cause sodium retention, so avoid its use in formulas for people with nervous system imbalances, cardiovascular imbalances, high or low blood pressure, or who are pregnant.

## Antispasmodic

For general pelvic spasms or cramps associated with urinary issues, consider wild yam, black haw, or cramp bark. For spasms of the ureter, urethra, or other urinary-specific spasm, consider corn silk.

## *Urinary Tract Formulas*
### A FORMULA FOR URINARY TRACT INFECTION WITH BURNING

› 2 parts cleavers

› 1 part garlic

› 1 part bearberry

› 1 part dandelion leaf

### A FORMULA FOR URINARY TRACT INFECTION WITH CRAMPS

› 2 parts calendula

› 1 part black haw

› 1 part cleavers

› 1 part corn silk

In addition to the above formulas, a helpful protocol will include dietary recommendations. A healthy diet is key in mitigating infection and pain in the urinary system. The guidelines are simple: reduce inflammatory foods (such as the nightshade family) and reduce calcifying foods (such as spinach, wood sorrel, and even chocolate). Greatly increase the amount of water drunk, being sure to take in a full six to eight glasses of distilled water daily.

Dietary changes, herbal formulary, and a healthy exercise schedule can support urinary health. Support your client with common sense and the herbs listed here based on their actions and effective use through many years of tradition.

# Endnote

Including plant medicines in your practice is one of the most rewarding ways to offer healing to your clients, and it allows you to be creative and versatile while using natural ingredients. As noted, there are many ways to create herbal formulary, and it is my hope that the structure outlined here gives you a solid foundation upon which to build blends that work effectively for you for years to come. As my students have told me, there are always more herbs to learn, but having this 4-tier formula as a basis allows them to "plug in" the right herbs regardless of the country, culture, or philosophy in which they are working. As you add more herbs to your repertoire, use this structure to help you organize your thoughts and ultimately provide the best and most appropriate botanical remedies to your family, clients, and community.

As always, appreciate the plants, enjoy the process, and share what you learn.

# PART SIX

# Glossaries

The glossaries included here are intended to serve as a useful reference for the herbalist or healing arts professional who wishes to create herbal formulas for a wide variety of conditions. Here you'll find a glossary of herbal actions (properties) that are commonly described in herbal medicine, as well as a "primer" in chemical constituents to give a general background as to the efficacy of herbs and their abilities to interact with the human body and mind. Additionally, two glossaries focus on tonics since the basis of herbal medicine is to support and nourish.

Please use common sense in your approach to plant medicine, understanding that specific drug-herb interactions and contraindications are beyond the scope of these glossaries. For drug-herb interactions, please consult with your trusted health care practitioner or knowledgeable pharmacist.

# Glossary A:
# Herbal Actions

Organizing herbs by their action (or effect on the body) has been one of the most popular ways to organize for my herb school students. It's a handy reference when you're looking for an herb based on what it does; for instance, is it nervine, which supports the nervous system as a tonic? Or is it astringent, meaning it is better used topically on the skin to tighten tissues during an infection? The action of the herb has been given a number of names by herbalists: the herb's virtue, its character, benefit, effect, property, etc. The action is what it does, not which body system it is most useful for. This is because actions overlap and can be used in various body systems. For instance, a spasmolytic (an herb that eases spasms) might be used for the digestive system as well as for arthritic muscles and joints.

For the purposes of glossary A and the individual profiles, *edible* refers to our ability to safely consume the plant or part of the plant as a normal and tasty table food, in salads, raw, or cooked. While many safe herbs make an acceptable tea or beverage, they are not necessarily edibles.

*Cerebral* refers to stimulant activity directed toward the brain, to distinguish it from nervine or nervous system actions. Also, though the skin is officially part of the integumentary system, sometimes it is categorically separated here so that *skin* refers to topical applications for surface issues while *integumentary* refers to topical or internal applications for muscle and deeper tissue complaints.

**Abortifacient:** Causes the abortion of a fetus during pregnancy. Multiple criteria cause an herb to be classed as an abortifacient: if it is emmenagogue (naturally stimulates the uterus and hormones to bring on the menstrual flow); if it is toxic or poisonous (such as pasqueflower); or if it acts as a vermifuge, stimulant, or strong purgative and stimulates any part of the body toward expulsion. Abortifacient herbs include pennyroyal, black walnut, tansy, blue cohosh. See oxytoxic.

**Adaptogen:** Supports the nervous system and helps the body and mind adapt to stress; supports our coping mechanisms; aid memory. Includes eleuthero, ginseng, vervain, skullcap, lemon balm, motherwort.

**Alterative:** Assists the body in proper elimination; traditionally used as "blood cleansers" or "springtime tonics." Generally used as hepatics to support and strengthen the liver and digestive system. Also called depurative. Includes dandelion, yellow dock, mustard greens, nettle, red clover.

**Anhidrotic:** An herb that suppresses sweating; antiperspirant.

**Analgesic** or **anodyne:** Pain-relieving. External or internal. Includes willow, meadowsweet, wintergreen, birch, lavender, chamomile, chickweed, hops, passionflower, poppy, St. John's wort, Jamaican dogwood.

**Anthelmintic:** Expels worms. See vermifuge.

**Antibiotic:** See antimicrobial.

**Anticatarrhal:** Acts as an astringent to dry up mucous secretions in the upper and lower respiratory tract. Includes elderflower, freeze-dried nettle root, goldenseal. Do not use during breastfeeding. See astringent.

**Antiemetic:** Relieves vomiting, stops spasms in the stomach and gut. Relieves nausea, such as travel sickness or morning sickness. Includes mint, ginger, chamomile, meadowsweet. See carminative.

**Anti-inflammatory:** Reduces inflammation in muscle tissues. Herbs for topical use include arnica, wintergreen, ginger, mustard, cayenne, Scotch pine, eucalyptus. Herbs for internal use include black cohosh, wild yam, raspberry, most of the carminative herbs.

**Antilithic:** Helps expel "gravel" or stones from the kidneys and bladder. Includes Joe Pye weed (gravel root), olive, corn silk, buchu, bearberry, usnea.

**Antimicrobial:** Either directly kills pathogens (parasites) in the body, or assists the body's immune defenses to kill them. Includes elderberry, elder flower, yarrow, garlic, cayenne, goldenseal, echinacea, gentian, myrrh, thyme, sage.

**Antineoplastic:** Neoplasm is cancer; antineoplastic herbs directly support the eradication of cancerous cells and tumors. Herbs undergoing clinical and laboratory study include red clover, barberry, and periwinkle.

**Antipruritic:** Reduces itching.

**Antispasmodic:** Directly affects muscle contractions; eases muscles, relieves soreness, stiffness, cramps, and spasms. Includes arnica (externally only), black cohosh, black haw, cramp bark, wild yam, valerian, skullcap, motherwort, lobelia. Synonym: spasmolytic.

**Antitussive:** Cough suppressant.

**Aperient:** See laxative.

**Aromatic:** Herbs composed of terpenes (essential oils) that produce fragrance. Aromatic herbs are often used as carminative herbs to expel gas and relieve indigestion.

**Astringent:** Tightens tissues both internally and externally. Acts as a styptic, dries up wet or weepy conditions. Use caution in breastfeeding as astringent herbs can dry up breast milk. Includes goldenseal, yarrow, parsley, oak, cranesbill, mullein, elecampane, sage, witch hazel.

**Anxiolytic:** Supports coping and relaxing mechanisms during stress and anxiety. Nervine tonic herbs that soothe the central nervous system without being sedative (soporific). Includes St. John's wort, vervain, lemon balm, motherwort, chamomile, skullcap.

**Bitter:** Herbs containing a wide variety of compounds that give a bitter taste. This taste stimulates the gastrointestinal tract and promotes the production of bile. Many bitters also help increase appetite, relieve nausea, and act as digestive tonics, though in the 4-tier formula they are seldom used as tier 1 tonics and instead are used as tier 3 corollary. Bitters include goldenseal, motherwort, yarrow, gentian, wild indigo, white horehound, calendula, chamomile, mugwort, wormwood, tansy, rue, walnut hull.

**Bronchial:** Respiratory herbs used to promote elimination of fluids and soothe the lung tissues. Some bronchial herbs are antispasmodic while others are expectorant.

**Carminative:** Aromatic herbs that soothe the muscles of the stomach and upper digestive tract. Full of volatile or essential oils (terpenes), carminative herbs relax the gastrointestinal tract and allow proper digestion to take place, often relieving gas pains, bloating, and digestive upset. Includes lemon balm, anise, licorice, ginger, mint, fennel, dill, lavender, coriander, cardamom, angelica, chamomile, caraway, cinnamon.

Cholagogue/Choleretic: Stimulates the production of bile from the gallbladder. Includes barberry, gentian, wild yam.

Contraindicated: An herb that should not be used with a particular over-the-counter or prescription medication. Some herbs will enhance a drug's effects while others will negate it, making dosages difficult or dangerous. Common examples of herbs that may be contraindicated with prescriptions (for a variety of illnesses) include St. John's wort, black pepper, parsley, nettles, hawthorn, and *echinacea*. Even relatively safe herbs and foods can interfere with prescription medication; for instance, garlic is often used to help reduce cholesterol, but it can increase the risk of bleeding if a person is taking Warfarin (also called Coumadin), which is an anticoagulant commonly taken to thin the blood and reduce the risk of embolism or thrombosis.[79] Therefore, garlic is contraindicated for people taking this drug. Contraindications are not limited to herbal medicines but they can also occur with foods (green leafy vegetables are contraindicated with patients taking Warfarin, too) and even other drugs or medications (patients on Warfarin are advised not to take NSAIDS).

Corrigent: An herb added to a formula to enhance flavor, for better tolerance. Spearmint and licorice are common corrigents.

---

79  Tachjian, Maria, and Jahangir (2010).

**Demulcent:** Soothing herbs (see mucilaginous) used internally for hot, sore, and inflamed conditions. Has a similar action to "emollients" that are used externally, but demulcent refers to internal relief. Includes comfrey, mallow, slippery elm, licorice, oats, lemon balm.

**Diaphoretic:** Promotes perspiration; sweating cools the skin and can help lower fevers (see Febrifuge). Generally these are circulatory stimulants. Includes cayenne, garlic, thyme, ginger, elder, black cohosh, yarrow.

**Diuretic:** Promotes the flow of urine through the kidneys and bladder. Many herbs, especially drunk cold, act as diuretics. Includes dandelion (also called *pis-en-lit*), yarrow, cleavers, parsley, corn silk, buchu, couchgrass.

**Emetic:** Causes vomiting and expulsion of contents from the stomach. In low doses, some are hallucinatory, while at higher doses they cause emesis. Includes ipecacuanha, lobelia, datura.

**Emmenagogue:** Herbs that bring on a late menstrual flow sometimes days or even weeks after the cycle is due. Can work through an endocrine action or a uterine-constricting action. Includes ginger, black cohosh, blue cohosh, moringa, pennyroyal. See abortifacient.

**Emollient:** Soothing to the skin. Cooling, moisturizing, hydrating. Includes calendula, lavender, oils of sweet almond and jojoba.

**Expectorant:** Causing fluids to be expelled from the lungs; useful in wet croupy coughs to help the lung muscle effectively purge itself of fluid. Includes pleurisy root, osha, peppermint.

**Febrifuge:** Helps to break or reduce fevers. Also called anti-pyretic. Includes yarrow, elderflower, elderberry, catnip, garlic, peppermint, boneset, thyme, cayenne.

**Galactagogue:** Promotes the secretion of breast milk in breastfeeding mothers. Helps during cases of stress or insufficient milk production. Includes blessed thistle, anise, caraway, fenugreek, milk thistle, fennel, dill, nettle.

**German Commission E:** the German equivalent of the United States Food and Drug Administration. Published "monographs" in the 1990s with extensive scientific reports about hundreds of medicinal herbs.

**Hemostatic:** See styptic.

**Hepatic:** Tones and supports the liver. Often high in iron, but not always. Hepatic herbs stimulate the production of bile and are traditionally used in "spring cleanses" or to support the liver after an illness or an addiction. Includes dandelion, yellow dock, turmeric, parsley, burdock. Hepatotoxic herbs are those that injure the liver.

**Homeopathic:** A philosophy of healing quite different from herbalism. Homeopathy was coined as a medical term by the German physician Samuel Hahnemann in 1807; he was dissatisfied with the dangers associated with modern medicine (especially bloodletting) and researched gentler methods. Homeopathy, which means "like cures like" and is opposite allopathy, or modern medicine, uses dilutions of animal parts, minerals, and plants. These dilutions affect an "energetic" response by the body, which is different from herbalism in which concentrates and extracts of plants (in water, honey, vinegar, or vodka, for instance) are used to support the body or organ system, or to directly kill a pathogen or support the immune system in eradicating illness.

**Inotropic:** Positive inotropic agents (including minerals, alkaloids, and esters) can increase the contractility of the heart muscle and are used to treat weakened heart conditions such as congestive heart failure, myocardial infarction, and cardiogenic shock. Digitalis is the best botanical example of a positively inotropic herb, with its chemical compound cardiac glycoside digoxin, along with those plants that contain the alkaloid berberine (including Oregon grape, barberry, and goldenseal). Negative inotropic agents are those that decrease the contractility of the heart muscle. Requires strong medical experience to use; not advocated in this book.

**Laxative:** Causes the bowels to loosen and expel feces; useful during constipation when there is no movement. Laxative herbs gently relax the muscles of the large intestine and the anus, allowing passage. Caution must be used against too much loss of water. Include senna, cascara sagrada, rhubarb root, yellow dock.

**Mucilaginous:** Of a slimy quality such that it brings relief to hot and inflamed conditions, either externally or internally. Cooling, soothing, gel-like. Include mallow, slippery elm, and plantain.

**Nervine:** Supports, tones, and/or nourishes the nervous system. Eases stress, anxiety, insomnia. Can be tier 1 herbs, used long-term. See anxiolytic.

**Nootropic:** An herb or drug used to enhance mental performance, particularly memory. Caffeine is nootropic, as are some amphetamines; their overuse can be dangerous. Herbs that are used to enhance cognitive performance include ginseng and ginkgo.

**Oxytocic:** Overly stimulating or even toxic to the uterus, such as pasqueflower. See abortifacient.

**Panacea:** Heal all; an agent that is assumed to cure anything and everything. A soother and comforter. Seventeenth century gardener John Evelyn used the term "catholicum" with much the same meaning.

**Pectoral:** See bronchial.

**Placebo:** An agent that cures without factual evidence of action but simply because the person believes it will cure them. Applied to herbal medicine, pharmaceutical (allopathic) medicine, and other therapies.

**Purgative:** Causes fluids to be expelled from any of the body's orifices: saliva, tears, urine, feces, vomit, sweat. Purgative herbs are highly irritating to the body and can be fatal in high doses. Purgatives include all diaphoretic herbs and all toxic herbs.

**Rubefacient:** Causes a reddening of the skin when rubbed topically (hence the root word *ruby*). Herbs such as fresh raw nettle are infamous for causing rashes and itching at the point of contact; they can be useful, though, because they bring fresh blood flow to the area, reduce inflammation, and relieve pain. The process of applying fresh raw nettles to sore joints and arthritic knuckles is known as "urtication," after nettle's Latin name *Urtica dioica*. Other rubefacients can include, depending on how they are used, cayenne, cinnamon, mustard.

**Sedative:** Promotes deep relaxation, and in some cases, sleep. Used to support the nervous system similar to anxiolytics, but with a stronger inhibitory action on energy and alertness. Mild sedatives include catnip, chamomile and wild lettuce. Stronger sedatives include kava kava, valerian, hops.

**Soporific:** Strong sedatives.

**Styptic:** Helps the body's defense mechanisms by ceasing blood flow to an area and forming scabs; a styptic applied to a topical wound will stop the bleeding. Efficient styptics include the astringent herbs yarrow, raspberry, oak.

**Tonic:** Supports a system or organ of the body either through nourishment (nutrients) or a toning and calming effect. Promotes vitality and strength, are extremely safe, and can be used long-term. Many body systems have tonics that are particularly suited to them, since many herbs seem to have an "affinity" for certain body systems. Respiratory tonics include mullein and licorice, skin tonics include calendula and rose, reproductive tonics include nettle and motherwort.

**Toxin:** A poisonous plant or part of a plant that creates an environment in which a body's organ or system can no longer function. In full herbal doses, toxins can be deadly; however, in carefully diluted doses used in homeopathy, certain toxic plants can be medicinal. Datura, belladonna, and henbane are examples of toxic herbs used in homeopathy.

**Vermifuge:** Expels worms. Usually extremely bitter herbs, these can be used topically or internally with great caution. Includes mugwort, walnut hull, cedar, juniper, wormwood, rue.

**Vulnerary:** Used topically to treat wounds. If you are vulnerable, you can be hurt. Many vulnerary herbs are traditionally used to "mend" broken skin and repair tissues, as well as kill germs and protect the site. Vulneraries include yarrow, plantain, calendula, mallow, comfrey, lavender, St. John's wort.

# Glossary B:
# Phytochemicals

Plants chemicals protect the plant from predation and encourage its reproduction and survival. Many of these ingredients also affect humans (and other mammals), and their use can be either toxic or nourishing. Botanical medicines are high in many phytochemicals that positively affect our heart rate, cardiovascular systems, immune system, ability to counter inflammation, and our ability to properly digest foods (to name just a few).

**acids, bases, and salts:** acids form hydrogen ions when dissolved in water, while a base produces hydroxyl ions in water. Salts form when an acid and a base combine.

**alkaloids:** Defined simply, alkaloids are organic nitrogenous compounds found in many plants and some animals. They are famous because of their marked physiological effects *not only on the body but also on the brain*. Most chemical compounds affect our bodies: they heal the skin or trigger an enzyme—but they do not have a noticeable impact on our brains, energy level, or clarity of thought. Tannins, for instance, astringe tissue but do not affect our brains. But bitter, water-soluble alkaloids do affect the mind, causing emotional, extra-sensory and nervous system reactions—sometimes good, sometimes not.

The word originated in the Arabic *al qualja*, meaning "ashes of plants," and most alkaloid names end in "-ine": nicotine, caffeine, mescaline, and berberine, for example. Nicotine is the chemical in tobacco responsible for not only relaxing muscle tissue but also calming the mind. Caffeine in *Theobroma* and coffee tenses the muscles, increases the heart rate, and propels the mind into over-alert hyperdrive. A single plant may possess two, three—or even a dozen—different alkaloids in any part of the plant: the seeds, fruits, leaves, stems, roots, rhizomes, or bark. They're even found in fungi.

Chemists ask the eternal question: Why do plants have alkaloids? An obvious answer might be for protection. A plant that produces a chemical that gives an animal a severe stomachache will discourage that animal from returning to eat more. But why would a plant cause an animal (or human) predator to have hallucinations? Or get the jitters? Or experience euphoria?

Alkaloids often become recreational drugs and can be toxic, killing animals and humans. A certain amount of quinine is effective against malaria (tertian fever) but too much monkshood can kill. A tincture of laudanum, with its high morphine and codeine content, can ease one into tranquility and lessen pain, but the dosage quickly becomes addictive and the patient's body debilitates rapidly.

But alkaloids show promise, as well. Berberine is an alkaloid found in many plants, most notably Chinese coptis and goldenseal. One study shows that in addition to being an antidiarrheal, antimicrobial, and anti-inflammatory, berberine may also support neuron health by inhibiting the amyloid-beta peptide that leads to Alzheimer's disease. [80]

**anthraquinones:** see quinones.

**bitter principles:** any chemical compound that produces a bitter flavor. Used in herbalism primarily for digestive upset and to address indigestion or loss of appetite.

**coumarins:** Coumarin is a naturally occurring, sweet-smelling chemical found in many plants and foods, including tonka beans, cinnamon, and sweet clover. Pharmaceutically, coumarin can be scientifically manipulated to create an anticoagulant (blood thinner) that is useful to combat hypertension and atherosclerosis; warfarin is the anticoagulant developed by the Wisconsin Alumni Research Foundation which has been branded under Coumadin and other names. [81] Though coumarin obtained from the South American tree tonka was used as a food flavoring early in the twentieth century, it can be hepatotoxic (toxic to the liver) and has been removed by the Food and Drug Administration as a flavoring agent and requires professional use in medical contexts. For these reasons, cinnamon and red clover may be herbal options for addressing hypertension, but should be avoided in people already taking anticoagulant drugs such as Warfarin (Coumadin).

**essential oils:** terpene molecules that provide the fragrance of a plant; also called volatile oils, meaning they readily evaporate and are not fixed. They may be formed by various mechanisms, including the hydrolysis of certain glycosides, and they occur in different plant parts in different species (petals, bark, leaves, hairs, etc.). Though

---

80   Asai, Iwata, and Yoshikawa (2007).

81   Claus and Tyler, Jr. (1965).

not entirely soluble in water, essential oils dissolve only enough to impart their fragrance to the water; they are however soluble in ether, alcohol, and most organic solvents.

**fats, lipids and oils:** carbon, hydrogen and low-oxygen esters formed by the reaction between an alcohol and an acid. Fats and fatlike substances are present in every living cell and are a principle kind of food substance.

**fatty acids:** formed by two principle groups (saturated and unsaturated). Examples of saturated fatty acids include those found in the plants laurel, coconut, cocoa, palm, and bayberry. Most fatty acids are unsaturated, such as those found in flax (also known as linseed).

**flavonoids (or bioflavonoids):** yellow polyphenolic compounds found in some plants including citrus, tea, wine, and dark chocolate. Much research indicates these compounds have an antioxidant effect and an anticancer (neoplastic) effect, while other research notes a carcinogenic potential. In vitro studies indicate anti-inflammatory and anticancer effects, with antioxidant properties possibly being the result of the body trying to rid itself of the substance through the urine. Quercetin is a type of flavonoid (a flavonol); anthocyanidins, and catechins are a subgroups. Single phenols are generally powerfully antiseptic and include salicylates (willow, *Salix* spp.) or eugenol (clove, *Eugenia caryophyllata*), while in the commercial laboratory phenols are transfigured into plastics, resins and nylon.

**glycosides:** There are many naturally occurring sugars: dextrose, fructose, glucose, sucrose, and lactose are the official sugars recognized by the U.S. Pharmacopeia and National Formulary (USP-NF). One or more sugars can be created when a glycoside compound is "hydrolyzed" or acted upon by an enzyme often found within the same plant but in different tissues. Glucose occurs most frequently.

Glycosides have profound affects upon the body; cardioactive glycosides, for example, affect the heart muscle by increasing its tone, exciting it, and causing it to contract. This can be useful for those with low blood pressure, as the glycoside will empower the heart by strengthening the pumping action. Strophanthus, squill, convallaria, and *Digitalis purpurea*, or foxglove, exhibit this action. *Digitalis's* dried leaf contains digitoxin, digoxin, and ouabain, among other powerful cardioactive glycosides. Many plants contain glycosides, including black mustard, wintergreen, and the laxatives senna and cascara sagrada.

**isoflavones:** produced primarily by the *Leguminoseae* (bean) family—particularly soy—isoflavones are antioxidant and in some cases anti-cancer. Isoflavones appear to have a strong estrogen-like effect.

**oleoresins:** combination of an oil and a resin. Softer than pure resins, called balsams.

**phospholipids:** highly complex fatty compounds that contain phosphorous; believed to assist with the permeability of protoplasmic membranes and with cell structure maintenance based on their emulsification properties.

**quinones:** quinones generally irritate a person, probably present in the plant for its own protection. Quinones are often colorful and many have been used as pigments or dyes: walnut contains juglone (the hull of the pod produces a dark greenish brown colorfast dye). There are several types of quinones: anthraquinones irritate the gastrointestinal tract, acting as purgatives. These include rhubarb and senna, two classic stimulators of the bowels that readily induce bowel movement and can be useful as laxatives during constipation. Other quinones include naphthaquinones and benzoquinones.

**resins:** a protective substance produced mainly by conifers; a viscous, sticky, and fragrant liquid comprised mainly of terpines. Insoluble in water but soluble in hot oils or alcohol.

**sterols:** alcohols, including cholesterol, highly prevalent in brain and nervous tissue. Animal tissues contain cholesterol while plant tissues contain phytosterols.

**tannins:** Typically, plants contain enzymes and proteins. Enzymes break proteins down into smaller particles, such as amino acids. Plants also contain tannins—these are astringent or antiseptic compounds that bring enzyme action to a screeching halt. Tannins restrict enzymes so they can't break down proteins. This is harmful for human digestion—think of black tea, for example, because the tannins in *Camellia sinensis* bind with living tissues and hamper proper digestion. (To avoid this, simply add milk to the tea, which negates the process.) When tannins are applied to living tissues, the action is called astringent because the tissues are "astringed" or tightened.

But tannins can be helpful to living tissues in the right circumstances. For instance, tannins can form a protective barrier under which new tissues can grow. Pharmacologist Varro Tyler gives the example of a burn patient: the exposed tissues of the burn contain proteins, and when tannins are introduced to these proteins, a protective (and antiseptic) coat is formed under which new tissue can regenerate. [82] Tannins can also be used as an antidote to toxic alkaloids, because the tannin will bind with the alkaloid to form an insoluble substance (a tannate), rendering those poisons ineffective.

The binding action of tannins is also useful for activities involving non-living tissue, such as "tanning" deerskin. When tannins bind with proteins to form a coat, they create a pliable

82   Claus and Tyler, Jr. (1965).

yet tough skin that is inherently preserved. Some scientists believe tannins are a waste product of the plant, because tannins are often found in the leaves of deciduous trees and, by falling off, will rid the plant of excess toxic tannins. Some of the many plants used medicinally for their tannins include:

- **witch hazel** (*Hamamelis virginiana*) leaf and twig. Astringent, hemostatic.

- **oak** (*Quercus* spp.) leaf, twig, acorn. Nutgall from Asia Minor is the result of an insect depositing its larvae in a mass on the oak tree's leaves. The gall contains a great deal of tannin. Known to Greeks since 450 BCE, the nutgall is a chief source of tannic acid.

- **New Jersey tea/red root** (*Ceanothus*) leaves, root. This was a tea substitute for Colonists during the Revolutionary War. Considered potent blood-coagulators.

- **cranesbill** (*Geranium maculatum*) root. Styptic, hemostatic, vulnerary. Contains gallic acid, similar to roses. These tiny roots are a traditional remedy for diarrhea and internal bleeding. They are taken internally (as a douche or tincture) or externally (as a poultice or compress).

- **rose** (*Rosa* spp.) petals and leaves. Harvested (especially from southern France and Morocco) for their mild tannic and gallic acid content. "Gallic" is from *Rosa gallica*, meaning "of Gaul," or France.

- **raspberry** (*Rubus idaeus*) and blackberry (*R. villosus*) root.

- **hemlock tree** (*Tsuga canadensis* and other spp.) bark.

- **India tree/kino** (*Pterocarpus marsupium*) astringent red juice from trunk of tree. Collectors make an incision in the trunk to collect the juice, which is dried in shallow pans in the sun. Once dried, the drug is shipped from Bombay; the preparation shipped from Madras is known as Malabar Kino.

**terpenes:** the chief component of resin, found most frequently in conifers and pines. Steroids derive from terpenes, as do many other chemical compounds from the oxidation of terpene hydrocarbons, including alcohols, aldehydes, ketones, phenols, phenolic ethers, esters, and oxides. Terpenes are the chief "ingredient" in essential oils.

**waxes:** fatty acid esters of saturated alcohols or sterols. They coat the outer surface of epidermal cell walls in plants to prevent water loss.

# Glossary C:
# Herbal Tonics

Because tonics are fundamental to herbal practice and to the 4-tier formula philosophy, this glossary lists tonic herbs individually, providing their names, indications, contra-indications, and a list of their dominant vitamins, minerals, and other phytochemicals. You'll also see which herbs they traditionally combine with as well as if the herb is edible or not, which is useful since tonics are meant to be taken long-term and if they can be a food, so much the better. The next glossary (glossary D) lists tonics organized by body system.

**ashwagandha,** *Withania somnifera*
>   **Best taken as:** capsule, powder, infusion, tincture
>   **Indicated for:** nervous disability, insomnia, nervous tension, anxiety, hypertension, exhaustion, inflammation

**Contraindications:** pregnancy (the American Herbal Products Association advises against its use during pregnancy, while it is still traditionally used in Ayurvedic medicine during pregnancy.) [83]

**Combines well with:** gotu kola, oatstraw, vervain, ginkgo

**burdock root,** *Arctium lappa*

**Best taken as:** infusion, vinegar tincture, powder, food

**Indicated for:** the liver, digestive system, skin, healthy hair and nails, bone health, as a springtime "blood cleanser"

**Contains:** vitamin C, calcium, iron, zinc

**Combines well with:** dandelion, yellow dock, chickweed

**chamomile,** *Matricaria recutita*

**Best taken as:** infusion, capsule, powder

**Indicated for:** the nervous system, the digestive system, muscles, and inflammation

**Contraindicated in:** severe depression, hay fever

**High in:** calcium, iron, magnesium, zinc

**Combines well with:** skullcap, vervain, lemon balm, hops, catnip, valerian

**comfrey leaf,** *Symphytum officinale*

**Best taken as:** infusion, capsule, powder, ointment

**Indicated for:** strong bones, hair and nails, elimination system, healthy skin

**Contraindications:** can cause stomach upset; root contains the hepatotoxic pyrrolizidine alkaloid. Use leaf internally in small amounts.

**Combines well with:** horsetail, oatstraw, raspberry leaf

---

83   Romm (2010).

**dandelion leaf** or **root,** *Taraxacum officinale*

    **Best taken as:** infusion, capsule, salad, granulated drink

    **Indicated for:** elimination system, strong hair and nails, healthy skin, circulatory system, reproductive system

    **Contraindications:** renal upset or failure, bladder stress, kidney stress, pregnancy (in high doses)

    **High in:** potassium, calcium, iron, magnesium, zinc, phosphorous, vitamins A, C, K, omega 3 fatty acids, omega 6 fatty acids

    **Combines well with:** yellow dock, burdock, milk thistle, nettle

**ginkgo,** *Ginkgo biloba*

    **Best taken as:** infusion, capsule, powder

    **Indicated for:** circulatory/vascular, the brain and mental function, stress and anxiety

    **Contraindications:** none

    **Combines well with:** gotu kola, lemon balm, oatstraw

**hawthorn berry, leaf,** and **flower,** *Cretaegus* spp.

    **Best taken as:** infusion, capsule, jam

    **Indicated for:** cardiovascular system, brain and mental function, respiratory system

    **Contraindicated in:** hypotension

    **High in:** calcium (berry), iron (berry), magnesium (berry)

    **Combines well with:** ginkgo, oatstraw, motherwort

**horsetail,** *Equisetum arvense*

    **Best taken as:** infusion, capsule, tincture

    **Indicated for:** musculoskeletal generation, bone repair, hair and skin, chronic bedwetting, prostate enlargement, kidney stones

    **Contraindicated in:** bone spurs, cigarette addiction, hypercalcemia, deficiency of vitamin B1, gout

    **High in:** silica

    **Combines well with:** comfrey leaf, oatstraw, cleavers, pipsissewa

**kelp,** *Laminaria* spp. and *Hijiki*

Best taken as: capsule, powder, food

Indicated for: tonic for strong hair, skin, bones, healthy liver

Contraindicated in: hyperthyroidism

High in: zinc, vitamins A and C, calcium, phosphorus, potassium, iron, magnesium.

Combines well with: burdock root

Note: use in small amounts due to high sodium content

**lemon balm,** *Melissa officinalis*

Best taken as: infusion, capsule, powder

Indicated for: brain and mental function, nerves, skin, digestive system, hyperthyroidism

Contraindicated in: hypothyroidism in large doses

High in: flavonoids, which can have an antioxidant effect, tannins, essential oil

Combines well with: vervain, oatstraw, nettle

**motherwort,** *Leonurus cardiaca*

Best taken as: tincture, capsule, powder

Indicated for: the nervous, digestive, reproductive, and cardiovascular systems

Contraindicated in: extreme hypotension, gastric or peptic ulcers, pregnancy

Combines well with: ginkgo, hawthorn, lemon balm

**nettle,** *Urtica dioica*

Best taken as: infusion, capsule, powder

Indicated for: skin, elimination system, reproductive system, pregnancy, breastfeeding, allergies, hair and nails, energy and stamina

Contraindicated in: diarrhea

**High in:** vitamin C, potassium, calcium, iron, magnesium, zinc
**Combines well with:** alfalfa, oatstraw, lemon balm

**oatstraw,** *Avena sativa*
    **Best taken as:** infusion, capsule, powder
    **Indicated for:** brain and mental function, nervous system, skin, bones, hair and nails
    **Contraindications:** none; widely regarded as safe.
    **High in:** vitamin C, calcium, iron, magnesium
    **Combines well with:** all herbs

**raspberry,** *Rubus idaeus*
    **Best taken as:** infusion, capsule
    **Indicated for:** women's reproductive system, uterine strength, strong hair, skin and bones
    **Contraindicated in:** breastfeeding (in large doses)
    **High in:** calcium, vitamin C, iron, magnesium
    **Combines well with:** mullein leaf, oatstraw, lemon balm, nettle, cranesbill

**rose petal,** *Rosa* spp.
    **Best taken as:** infusion, capsule, powder, jam; topically as a spray or oil
    **Indicated for:** grief, depression, uncertainty, confusion, over-heated conditions, hypertension, hyperthyroid, mental debility, anger
    **Contraindications:** none
    **Combines well with:** oatstraw, violet, nettle, ashwagandha, motherwort

**saw palmetto,** *Serenoa repens*
    **Best taken as:** infusion, capsule, tincture; short-term use is best
    **Indicated for:** prostate gland in men, dysmenorrhea, reproductive debility

Contraindicated in: pregnancy, breastfeeding, possibly with previous
   heart attack
Combines well with: green tea, nettle root, hydrangea

violet flower and leaf, *Viola odorata*
   Best taken as: infusion, capsule, food
   Indicated for: nervous, digestive, respiratory and reproductive
      systems; healthy skin, hair, and nails; inflammation;
   Contraindications: none
   Contains: leaf is high in vitamin C, calcium
   Combines well with: self heal, chickweed, burdock root, nettle,
      mint

# Glossary D:
# Herbal Tonics by Body System

Organizing tonic herbs by body system is a useful way to reference about them. This glossary makes for a quick guide when searching for the right tonic herb to use as support or nourishment for a given body system. Please refer to this list as a basis and add other herbs as you become familiar with them for certain conditions within a body system. Please remember that there are contraindications to some herbs; for instance, while St. John's wort is listed as a tonic herb under "nervous system," because of its influence on serotonin it may be contraindicated for someone taking MAOI medication. Choose another tonic herb from the list if in doubt. Keep in mind, also, that some of these are tier 2 Specifics and may be too strong.

**Endocrine System**
    burdock
    cleavers
    echinacea

dandelion

red clover

yellow dock

bladderwrack

bugleweed

eleuthero

licorice

wild yam

## Nervous System

oats

eleuthero

skullcap

chamomile

vervain

ginkgo

St. John's wort

ashwagandha

lemon balm

rose

borage

wild lettuce

rhodiola

## Musculoskeletal System

horsetail

oats

comfrey leaf

chickweed

nettle

ashwagandha

## Cardiovascular System

hawthorn

bugleweed

motherwort

borage

rose

linden

ginkgo

## Reproductive System

*Women's hormone tonics*

red clover

black cohosh

chaste tree berry

angelica

saw palmetto berry

nettle

eleuthero

*Uterine tonics*

raspberry leaf

partridgeberry herb

blue cohosh root

helonias (false unicorn root)

nettle

*Men's hormone tonics*

eleuthero

panax ginseng

saw palmetto

green tea

**Digestive System**

dill

fennel

spearmint

catnip

chamomile

ginger (in small doses)

dandelion

linden

**Detoxification/Elimination System**

*Hepatic tonics*

dandelion root and leaf

motherwort

hops

milk thistle

blessed thistle

ginger in small doses

*Lymph tonics*

cleavers

calendula

echinacea

*Urinary tonics*

corn silk

dandelion leaf

bearberry

violet

yarrow

motherwort (in small doses)

slippery elm

## Respiratory System

mullein

coltsfoot

elecampane

elderflower

## Immune System

calendula

cleavers

garlic

red clover

elderberry

boneset

elderflower

burdock root

ginkgo

nettle

lemon balm

spearmint

rose hips

mushrooms, including reishi

# Glossary E:
# United Plant Savers Lists

You will have noticed that this book includes some herbs that are, in their wild habitats, threatened or in danger of becoming overharvested. I include them here because they are effective medicines, but I preface their use with a note about their conservation, because to use them recklessly, especially in a commercial environment, will surely lead to their extinction.

Many of these herbs are common in historic herbal treatments for midwives and women and for a wide range of health issues for people of all ages, and they are in precipitous decline thanks to overharvesting, sensitivity, and widespread habitat destruction. In my years in the mountains of Southern Appalachia, I found a number of secluded and shady hillsides brimming with trillium blossoms and lady's slipper, but only in a few wild places did I find false unicorn root, and only once did I come across wild black cohosh. Ginseng is rare enough to elicit cries of joy when found in the forest. I met many old-timers who expressed surprise at the decline of these valuable herbs, saying they remember picking lady's slippers by the basketful when they were young. Combine that free-for-all harvesting with today's rampant house-building and fragile habitat loss and it's no surprise these medicinal herbs are in great decline.

The conversation about continued use of these plants is interesting and important: knowing that these plants are at-risk of becoming endangered, should the herbalist or healing arts practitioner harvest them? Use them? Sell them? Completely ceasing activity with these plants may very well help secure their future existence, but it is also important to continue limited and respectful use of our inherited traditions, safeguarding the knowledge of their medicinal actions and preserving our understanding of their use in our medical repertoire. It is a fine line to walk and must be undertaken with care, respect, and a certain restraint.

The United Plant Savers (UpS) is a commendable organization that exists to protect native medicinal plants of the United States and Canada and their native habitat while ensuring an abundant renewable supply of medicinal plants for the future. In addition to their research, educational, and conservational activities and services, this member-driven organization produces two valuable lists to guide harvesters, growers, herbal craftspeople, retailers, and health practitioners in their selection and use of medicinal plants. Their list criteria are based on various factors, including the life span of the plant and its reproductive processes, the effects of over-harvest on the plant, its natural abundance and range, its habitat vulnerability and threats to its survival, and commercial factors such as market demand, yield, and whether it cultivates easily or not. Rather than pursuing a moratorium on the use of these plants, UpS is initiating programs to conserve them.

In an effort to promote this non-profit organization (of which I am a member) and to help the reader decide whether to use any of these plants in a formula, I am including the two lists they publish—the "At-Risk" list and the "To-Watch" list, both reprinted here with permission. Please visit their website to learn more: http://www.unitedplantsavers.org

# UpS At-Risk List

- **american ginseng,** *Panax quinquefolius*
- **bloodroot,** *Sanguinaria canadensis*
- **black cohosh,** *Actaea racemosa L.*
- **blue cohosh,** *Caulophyllum thalictroides*
- **echinacea,** *Echinacea* spp.
- **eyebright,** *Euphrasia* spp.
- **false unicorn root** (helonias), *Chamaelirium luteum*
- **goldenseal,** *Hydrastis canadensis*
- **lady's slipper orchid,** *Cypripedium* spp.
- **lomatium,** *Lomatium dissectum*
- **osha,** *Ligusticum porterii, L.* spp.
- **peyote,** *Lophophora williamsii*
- **sandalwood,** *Santalum* spp. (Hawaii only)
- **slippery elm,** *Ulmus rubra Sundew, Drosera* spp.
- **trillium** or **beth root,** *Trillium* spp.
- **true unicorn,** *Aletris farinose*
- **venus fly trap,** *Dionaea muscipula*
- **Virginia snakeroot,** *Aristolochia serpentaria*
- **wild yam,** *Dioscorea villosa, D.* spp.

# UpS To Watch List

- arnica, *Arnica* spp.

- butterfly weed (pleurisy root), *Asclepias tuberosa*

- cascara sagrada, *Frangula purshiana*

- chaparro, *Casatela emoryi*

- elephant tree, *Bursera microphylla*

- gentian, *Gentiana* spp.

- goldthread (coptis), *Coptis* spp.

- kava kava, *Piper methysticum* (Hawaii only)

- lobelia, *Lobelia* spp.

- maidenhair fern, *Adiantum pendatum*

- mayapple, *Podophyllum peltatum*

- Oregon grape, *Mahonia* spp.

- partridgeberry, *Mitchella repens*

- pink root, *Spigelia marilandica*

- pipsissewa, *Chimaphila umbellata*

- ramps, *Allium tricoccum*

- spikenard, *Aralia racemosa, A. californica*

- stone root, *Collinsonia canadensis*

- stream orchid, *Epipactis gigantea*

- turkey corn, *Dicentra canadensis*

- white sage, *Salvia apiana*

- wild indigo, *Baptisia tinctoria*

- yerba mansa, *Anemopsis californica*

# Bibliography

Alzheimer's Association. "What is Alzheimer's?" *Alz.org.* 2016. http://www
.alz.org/alzheimers_disease_what_is_alzheimers.asp.

Ambegaokar, SS, L. Wu, K. Alamshahi, and J. Lau. "Curcumin inhibits
dose-dependently and time-dependently neuroglial cell proliferation
and growth." *Neuroendocrinology Letters* 24, no. 6 (Dec 2003): 469–73.

American Botanical Council. "The Commission E Monographs/
Lemon Balm." *American Botanical Council.* March 1990. http://cms
.herbalgram.org/commissione/Monographs/Monograph0225.html
(accessed November 2016).

American Chemical Society. "Researchers call herbs rich source of
healthy antioxidants; Oregano ranks highest." *Science Daily.* 01 2002.
https://www.sciencedaily.com/releases/2002/01/020108075158.htm.

Asai, Masashi, N. Iwata, and A. Yoshikawa. "Berberine alters the
processing of Alzheimer's amyloid precursor protein to decrease AB
secretion." *Biochemical and Biophysical Research Communications* 352,
no. 2 (Jan 2007): 498–502.

Behall, Kay, and Judith Hallfrisch. "Oats as a Functional Food for Health." *United States Department of Agriculture.* November. 16, 2006. https://www.ars.usda.gov/research/publications/publication /?seqNo115=181785&pf=1.

Bellebuono, Holly. *Women Healers of the World: The Traditions, History & Geography of Herbal Medicine.* New York: Helios Press, Skyhorse Publishing Inc., 2014.

Bliss, Rosalie Marion. "Study Shows Consuming Hibiscus Tea Lowers Blood Pressure." *United States Department of Agriculture, Agricultural Research Service.* November 10, 2008. https://www.ars.usda.gov/news -events/news/research-news/2008/study-shows-consuming-hibiscus -tea-lowers-blood-pressure/.

———. "Study Shows Tea Consumption Lowers Blood Cholesterol." *United States Department of Agriculture, Agricultural Research Service.* September 30, 2003. https://www.ars.usda.gov/news -events/news/research-news/2003/study-shows-tea-consumption -lowers-blood-cholesterol/.

Buhner, Stephen Harrod. *Healing Lyme: Natural Healing and Prevention of Lyme Borreliosis and Its Coinfections.* Silver City, NM: Raven Press, 2005.

———. *Herbal Antibiotics: Natural Alternatives for Treating Drug-Resistant Bacteria.* North Adams, MA: Storey Publishing, 1999.

Cabrera, Chanchal. ""Building a Formula—Selection Criteria and Dosing Strategies." July 7, 2012. http://www.chanchalcabrera.com /building-a-formula/.

"Cardiovascular Diseases (CVDs)." World Health Organization. September 2016. http://www.who.int/mediacentre/factsheets/fs317=/en/.

Castleman, Michael. *The New Healing Herbs: The Classic Guide to Nature's Best Medicines.* New York: Rodale, 2001.

Clare, Bevin. "Herbs and the Immune System." Black Mountain, NC: Southeast Wise Women Herbal Conference, October 2012.

Claus, Edward P., and Varro E. Tyler, Jr. *Pharmacognosy.* 5th. Philadelphia, PA: Lea & Febiger, 1965.

Craft, Suzanne, Jessica Freiherr, and Manfred Hallschmid. "Intranasal Insulin as a Treatment for Alzheimer's Diease: A Review of the Basic Research and Clinical Evidence." *CNS Drugs* 27, no. 7 (Jul 2013): 505–514.

Dalley, Stephanie. *Myths from Mesopotamia: Creation, the Flood, Gilgamesh, and Others.* New York: Oxford University Press, 2008.

Deisseroth, Karl. "A Look Inside the Brain." *Scientific American* 315 (October 2016).

DelaPena, Auntie Velma, interview by Holly Bellebuono. Waimanalo, HI (February 3, 2009).

Dierman, D. Van, A. Marston, and J. Bravo. "Monoamine oxidase inhibition by Rhodiola rosea L. roots." *Journal of Ethnopharmacology* 122, no. 2 (March 2009): 397–401.

Doidge, Norman. *The Brain's Way of Healing: Remarkable Discoveries and Recoveries From the Frontiers of Neuroplasticity.* NY: Viking /Penguin Group, 2015.

Foster, Steven, and James Duke. *Eastern/Central Medicinal Plants and Herbs.* NY: Peterson Field Guides/Houghton-Mifflin, 2000.

Frydman-Marom, Anat, Aviad Levin, and Dorit Farfara. "Orally administered cinnamon extract reduces Beta Amyloid Oligomerization and corrects cognitive impairment in Alzheimer's Disease animal models." *Public Library of Science*, January 2011.

Galen. *On the Natural Faculties.* Translated by Arthur John Brock. Cambridge, MA: Harvard University Press, 1952.

Gilday, Kate. "An Herbal Approach to Lyme and Possible Co-Infections." *Celebrating the Healing Power of Plants.* Wheaton College, MA: The International Herb Symposium, 2013. 90–95.

Gladstar, Rosemary. *Herbal Healing for Women: Simple Home Remedies for Women of All Ages.* NY: Fireside, 1993.

Grieve, Maude. *A Modern Herbal.* New York, NY: Dover Publications Inc., 1971.

Herraiz, T., D. Gonzalez, C. Ancin-Azpilicueta, VJ Aran, and H. Guillen. "Food and Chemical Toxicology." *NCBI National Institutes of Health.* March 2010. https://www.ncbi.nlm.nih.gov/pubmed/200 36304?itool=EntrezSystem2.PEntrez.Pubmed.Pubmed_ResultsPanel .Pubmed_RVDocSum&ordinalpos=1.

Hoffmann, David. *Therapeutic Herbalism: A Correspondence Course.* Santa Barbara, CA, 1996.

———. *Healthy Digestion: A Natural Approach to Relieving Indigestion, Gas, Heartburn, Constipation, Colitis, and More.* Pownal, VT: Storey Books, 2000.

Hui, Hongxiang, George Tang, and Vay Liang W. Go. "Hypoglycemic herbs and their action mechanisms." *Chinese Medicine Journal, BioMed Central.* June 12, 2009. https://cmjournal.biomedcentral. com/articles/10.1186/1749-8546-4-11.

Johnson, Jeremy. "Carnosol: A Promising Anti-Cancer and Anti-Inflammatory Agent." *Cancer Letters* (Elsevier) 305, no. 1 (June 2011).

Jordan, Michael. *The Green Mantle: An Investigation Into Our Lost Knowledge of Plants.* London: Cassell & Co., 2001.

Jumbo-Lucioni, Patricia. "Curcumin's ability to fight Alzheimer's studied." Vanderbilt University. Jan 8, 2015. https://news.vanderbilt.edu/2015/01/08/curcumin's-ability-to-fight-alzheimer-studied/.

Kalb, Rosalind C. *Multiple Sclerosis: The Questions You Have the Answers You Need.* NY: Demos Health Books, 2012.

Karaberopoulos, Demetrios, and Marianna Karamanou. "The theriac in antiquity." *The Lancet* 379, no. 9830 (May 2012): 1942–1943.

Kartalis, A., M. Didagelos, and I. Georgiadis. "Effects of Chios mastic gum on cholesterol and glucose levels of healthy volunteers." *European Journal of Preventive Cardiology* 23, no. 7 (May 2016): 722–729.

Katrina I. Makris. *Out of the Woods: Healing Lyme Disease—Body, Mind & Spirit.* Santa Rosa, CA: Elite Books, 2011.

Katzenschlager, R., A. Evans, and A. Manson. "Mucuna pruriens in Parkinson's Disease: a double blind clinical and pharmacological study." *Journal of Neurology, Neurosurgery and Psychiatry* (BMJ Group) 75, no. 12 (December 2004).

Keay, John. *The Spice Route: A History.* Berkeley, CA: University of California Press, 2006.

Kloss, Jethro. *Back to Eden.* Kloss Family Heirloom Edition. Loma Linda, CA: Back to Eden Books, 1982.

Krawitz, C., MA Mraheil, and M. Stein. "Inhibitory activity of a standardized elderberry liquid extract against clinically-relevant human respiratory bacterial pathogens and influenza A and B viruses." *BMC Complementary and Alternative Medicine Journal* 11, no. 16 (Feb 2011).

Levy, Juliette de Bairacli. *Herbal Handbook for Everyone.* London: Faber and Faber Limited, 1966.

Lewis, Zoe A. *I Hope They Know: The Essential Handbook on Alzheimer's Disease and Care.* College Station, TX: Virtualbookworm.com Publishing Inc., 2008.

Lin, Liang-Tzung, Hsu Wen-Chan, and Lin Chun-Ching. "Antiviral Natural Products and Herbal Medicines." *Journal of Traditional and Complementary Medicine* 4(1) (Jan-Mar 2014): 24-35.

Low Dog, Tieraona. "A Common Sense Approach to Attention Deficit Hyperactive Disorder." *Exploring Nature's Pharmacy.* Black Mountain, NC: Medicines from the Earth, 1997.

McIntyre, Anne. "Rasayana: The Ayurvedic Path to Rejuvenation." *Celebrating the Healing Power of Plants.* Wheaton, MA: The International Herb Symposium, 2013. 239-243.

Mishra, S., and K. Palanivelu. "NCBI National Institutes of Health." *PubMed.gov.* January 11, 2008. https://www.ncbi.nlm.nih.gov /pubmed/19966973.

Monte, Suzanne De La, and Jack Wands. "Alzheimer's Disease is Type 3 Diabetes—Evidence Reviewed." *Journal of Diabetes and Science Technology* 2, no. 6 (Nov. 2008): 1101–1113.

Moore, Donnica. *Women's Health for Life: Written by Women for Women: Symptoms, Treatment, Prevention.* New York, NY: Dorling Kindersley, 2009.

Natarajan, C., and John Bright. "Curcumin inhibits experimental allergic Encephalomyelitis by Blocking IL-12 Signaling." *Journal of Immunology* 168, no. 12 (June 2002).

National Institute on Aging. "Alzheimer's Disease Genetics Fact Sheet." *NIH National Institute on Aging.* U.S. Department of Health and Human Services. October 20, 2016. https://www.nia.nih.gov /alzheimers/publication/alzheimers-disease-genetics-fact-sheet.

Mitchell, William. "Botanial Management of Alzheimer's and Parkinson's Diseases." In *Medicines From the Earth: Exploring Nature's Pharmacy*, by Gaia Herbal Research Institute. Black Mountain, NC, 1997.

Nizet, Viktor, and Marc Rothenberg. "Mitochondrial Missile Defense." *Nature Medicine* 14 (2008): 910–912.

Orr, Stephen. *The New American Herbal*. New York, NY: Clarkson Potter Publishers/Random House, 2014.

Panossian, Alexander, and George Wikman. "Pharmacology of Schisandra chinensis Bail: An Overview of Russian research and uses in medicine." *Journal of Ethnopharmacology* (Elsevier) 118, no. 2 (July 2008): 183–212.

Park, Byeoung-Soo, Lee Hyun-Kyung, and Lee Sung-Eun. "Antibacterial activity of Tabebuia impetiginosa Martius ex DC (Taheebo) against Helicobacter pylori." *Journal of Ethnopharmacology* (Elsevier) 105, no. 1–2 (April 2006): 255–262.

Patnaik, Naveen. *The Garden of Life: An Introduction to the Healing Plants of India*. NY: Doubleday, 1993.

Peters, David, and Kenneth R. Pelletier. *New Medicine: Complete Family Health Guide*. NY: Dorling Kindersley, 2005.

Phaneuf, Holly. *Herbs Demystified: A Scientist Explains How the Most Common Herbal Remedies Really Work*. NY: Marlowe & Company, 2005.

Robertsdottir, Anna Rosa. "Medicinal Plants of Iceland." *Celebrating the Healing Power of Plants*. Wheaton, MA: The International Herb Symposium, 2013.

Romm, Aviva. *Botanical Medicine for Women's Health*. St. Louis, MO: Churchill Livingstone Elsevier, 2010.

Romm, Aviva, and Tracy Romm. *ADHD Alternatives: A Natural Approach to Treating Attention-Deficit Hyperactivity Disorder.* Pownal, VT: Storey Books, 2000.

Sanders, Jack. *The Secrets of Wildflowers: A Delightful Feast of Little-Known Facts, Folklore and History.* Guilford, CT: The Lyons Press, 2003.

Shrikant, Mishra, and Kalpana Palanivelu. "The effect of curcumin (turmeric) on Alzheimer's disease: An overview." *Annals of Indian Academy of Neurology* 11, no. 1 (Jan–Mar 2008): 13–19.

Skugor, Mario. *The Cleveland Clinic Guide to Thyroid Disorders.* NY: Kaplan Publishing, 2009.

"Smoking and Tobacco Use. Highlights: Smoking Among Adults in the United States: Coronary Heart Disease and Stroke." *Centers for Disease Control and Prevention.* 2004. http://www.cdc.gov /tobacco/data_statistics/sgr/2004/highlights/heart_disease/index .htm.

Stamets, Paul. "Mushrooms and Mycelium Help the Microbiome." *Fungi Perfecti.* October 2015. http://www.fungi.com/blog/items /microbiome.html.

Stansberry, Jill, and Terry Willard. "Q&A: Antimicrobial Herbs for Lyme Disease Treatment." *Mother Earth Living,* March/April 2002.

Stearn, William. *Stearn's Dictionary of Plant Names for Gardeners: A Handbook on the Origin and Meaning of Botanical Names of Some Cultivate Plants.* Portlant, OR: Timber Press, 2002.

Stevenson, Daniel C, and Massachusetts Institute of Technology. *The Internet Classics Archive: 441 searchable works of classical literature.* 2001. Archived Web Site. Retrieved from the Library of Congress, https ://www.loc.gov/item/lcwa00095452/.

Stone, Merlin. *When God Was A Woman.* NY: Barnes & Noble Inc., 1976.

Storl, Wolf D. *Healing Lyme Disease Naturally.* Berkeley, CA: North Atlantic Books, 2010.

Tachjian, A., V. Maria, and A. Jahangir. "Use of Herbal Products and Potential Interactions in Patients With Cardiovascular Diseases." *Journal of the American College of Cardiology*, 55(6), 515–525, 2010. http://doi.org/10.1016/j.jacc.2009.07.074.

The Center for Integrative Medicine at Duke University. *The Duke Encyclopedia of New Medicine.* London: Rodale Books International, 2006.

Thompson Healthcare Inc. *PDR for Herbal Medicines.* 4th Edition. Montvale, NJ: Thompson Healthcare Inc., 2007.

Tierra, Michael. *The Way of Herbs.* NY: Pocket Books, 1990.

Varro, Tyler E. *The Honest Herbal: A Sensible Guide to the Use of Herbs and Related Remedies.* 3rd. NY: Pharmaceutical Products Press.

Weil, Andrew. *Healthy Aging: A Lifelong Guide to Your Physical and Spiritual Well-Being.* NY: Knopf, 2005.

Wheatley, David. "Safety of St. John's wort (Hypericum perforatum)." *The Lancet* 355, no. 9203 (February 2000): 576.

Wiesman, Janice F. *Peripheral Neuropathy: What It Is and What You Can Do To Feel Better.* Baltimore, MD: Johns Hopkins University Press, 2016.

Winston, David. "Adaptogens: Herbs for Strength, Stamina, and Stress Relief." *Celebrating the Healing Power of Plants.* Wheaton, MA: The International Herb Symposium, 2013. 414–419.

_____. "Differential Treatment of Depression and Anxiety with Botanical and Nutritional Medicines." *Celebrating the Healing Power of Plants.* Wheaton, MA: The International Herb Symposium, 2013. 405–413.

World Health Organization. "Nutrition: Micronutrient Deficiencies." *World Health Organization.* 2016. http://www.who.int/nutrition/topics/ida/en/.

Zhang, L., M. Fiala, J. Cashman, and J. Sayre. "Curcuminoids enhance amyloid-beta uptake by macrophages of Alzheimer's disease patients." *Journal of Alzheimer's Disease* 10, no. 1 (Sep 2006): 1–7.

# Index

alfalfa, 27, 35, 215, 223, 239, 317

*Allium sativum*
See garlic

aloe vera, 61, 62, 71, 72, 195, 197

*Aloysia citrodora*
See lemon verbena

alterative, 107, 108, 110, 191, 204, 224, 262, 296

Alzheimer's, 122, 127, 139, 141–147, 307

Amanda McQuade Crawford, 21

amenorrhea, 215–217, 235, 252

*Ammi visnaga*
See khella

amphoteric, 262

amyotrophic lateral sclerosis, 127

analgesic, 97, 101, 128, 178, 183, 184, 190, 193, 194, 197, 199, 216, 284, 296

androgen, 203, 279

andrographis, 173, 176

*Andrographis paniculata*
See andrographis

anemia, 33, 34, 220–222, 232

aneurism, 82, 90

angelica, 41, 68, 134, 183, 184, 216, 239, 252, 254, 299, 321

angina pectoris, 90, 92

anise, 20, 22, 68, 245, 299, 301

Anne McIntyre, 94

anovulation, 213–215, 235

anti-inflammatory, 60, 61, 63, 66, 68, 79, 102, 106, 110, 112, 113, 130, 156, 160, 166, 173, 174, 178, 179, 182–184, 190, 196, 197, 202, 203, 216, 218, 221, 225, 232, 239, 246, 253, 272, 273, 275, 284, 287, 297, 306, 308

antidepressant, 84, 131, 132, 135, 145, 265

antifungal, 102, 106, 156–158, 160, 186, 189, 204, 205

antimicrobial, 19, 67, 106, 110, 111, 113–115, 145, 157, 162, 165, 176, 205, 243, 246, 272, 273, 279, 283–286, 297, 306

antipruritic, 197, 297

antispasmodic, 60, 66, 79, 97, 105, 111, 113–115, 128, 158, 178, 179, 183, 216, 219, 220, 225, 229, 232, 283, 287, 298

antitussive, 112–114, 158, 298

antiviral, 103, 107, 131, 145, 156, 164–167, 174, 256

anxiety, 60, 68, 69, 80, 121, 128, 130, 131, 135, 139, 170, 178, 182, 198, 199, 201, 228, 229, 235, 240, 242, 251, 253, 255, 257, 267, 274, 298, 302, 313, 315

anxiolytic, 132, 139, 140, 166, 179, 214, 235, 247, 262, 263, 284, 298, 302, 303

*Apium graveolens*
See celery seed

*Apium petroselinum*
See parsley

*Aralia nudicaulis*
See wild sarsaparilla

*Arctium lappa*
See burdock

*Armoracia rusticana*
See horseradish

arnica, 41, 42, 178–181, 197, 246, 297, 328

arrowroot, 61

*Artemisia absinthium*
See wormwood

*Artemisia vulgare*
See mugwort

arthritis, 41, 42, 60, 103, 154, 177, 178, 180–182, 287

*Asclepias tuberosa*
See pleurisy root

ashwagandha, 27, 31, 95, 128, 131, 136, 214, 235, 236, 254, 256, 257, 262, 313, 317, 320

asthma, 110, 111, 114–116, 161, 169

astragalus, 31, 107, 112, 128, 129, 155, 167, 169, 172, 174, 176, 268 astringent, 28, 55, 67, 69, 70, 81, 84–86, 102, 105–107, 114, 115, 157, 160, 183, 188, 196, 203, 217, 221, 224, 232, 243, 245, 277, 283, 284, 286, 295, 297, 298, 304, 310–312

atherosclerosis, 74, 76, 86–88, 274, 275, 307

attention deficit hyperactivity disorder, 135, 136, 139

*Avena sativa*
  See oats

Ayurveda, 18, 30, 31, 61, 186, 278, 314

# B

bacopa, 145, 147

*Bacopa monnieri*
  See bacopa

barberry, 155, 172, 286, 297, 299, 302

basil, 94

bearberry, 39, 40, 285, 286, 288, 297, 322

belladonna, 304

benign prostatic hypertrophy, 272–274

*Berberis vulgaris*
  See barberry

birch, 42, 103, 296

bitter, 3, 19, 23, 31, 36–42, 54, 55, 60, 66, 67, 77, 79, 81, 83, 94, 97, 102, 107, 113, 129, 138, 144, 162, 166, 178, 183, 184, 190, 198, 201, 215, 217, 221, 233, 256, 262, 267, 275, 278, 286, 298, 304, 306, 307

black catechu, 70

black cohosh, 134, 183, 212, 214, 215, 217, 220, 225, 229, 230, 232, 235, 236, 241, 242, 252, 254, 255, 257, 297, 300, 321, 325, 327

black cumin, 189, 191, 202

black haw, 219, 220, 225, 231, 232, 287, 288, 297

black pepper, 147, 299

black tea, 85, 277, 310

black willow, 41

blackberry, 70, 311

bladderwrack, 29, 167, 214,
221, 233, 264, 266, 320

blessed thistle, 245, 301, 322

bloating, 49, 52, 59, 60, 63,
67–69, 71, 161, 225, 230,
231, 240, 251, 299

blue cohosh, 212, 241, 296,
300, 321, 327

bogbean, 42

boneset, 175, 300, 323

borage, 76, 92, 94, 232,
320, 321

boswellia, 61, 62

BPH
See benign prostatic
hypertrophy

bradycardia, 264

breast milk, 68, 102, 111, 173,
245, 247, 298, 301

breastfeeding, 102, 106, 111,
190, 243, 245–247, 297,
298, 301, 316–318

bronchitis, 110, 111, 114,
115, 169

buchu, 39, 297, 300

bugleweed, 214, 267, 320, 321

bupleurum, 55

*Bupleurum falcatum*
See bupleurum

burdock, 34, 56, 57, 191,
201, 204, 205, 224, 256,
268, 301, 314–316, 318,
319, 323

burns, 192–195, 197

C

calcium, 27, 33, 34, 63, 78, 80,
222, 223, 238, 239, 283,
314–318

*Camellia sinensis*
See black tea

cancer, 3, 32, 56, 61, 63, 108–
110, 112, 146, 153, 171,
172, 174, 190, 252, 264,
272, 273, 297

*Candida albicans*, 56, 65, 157,
159, 160, 187, 188

*Capsella bursa-pastoris*
See shepherd's purse

*Capsicum annuum*
See cayenne

*Chimaphila umbellata*
See pipsissewa

cholecystitis, 63

cholesterol, 77, 80, 82, 86–91,
108, 162, 204, 253,
299, 310

chronic obstructive pulmonary
disease (COPD), 75

chronic pelvic pain (CPP), 128,
182, 183

chronic stress, 104, 130, 131,
188, 278

cinnamate, 127

cinnamon, 31, 36, 41, 53, 68,
77, 86, 103, 127, 130,
146, 147, 159, 166,
180, 217, 254, 265,
299, 303, 307

cleavers, 40, 42, 56, 57, 103,
104, 107, 108, 172, 191,
204, 205, 224, 234, 266,
285, 286, 288, 300, 315,
319, 322, 323

clove, 27, 31, 34–36, 42, 101,
102, 106, 108, 157, 159,
167, 189, 192, 194, 195, 197,
199–201, 204, 205, 214, 215,
224, 235, 239, 242, 243, 252,
265, 268, 296, 297, 307, 308,
320, 321, 323

cocoa, 95, 139, 308

coffee, 58, 63, 221, 233, 306

colic, 58, 67, 68, 179, 245

*Collinsonia*
See stone root

coltsfoot, 113, 116, 323

comfrey, 34, 109, 115, 194, 196,
197, 200, 243, 300, 304,
314, 315, 320

constipation, 52, 56, 60, 61,
65–67, 71, 72, 96, 182,
218, 302, 309

cooling herbs, 16, 219, 224,
254, 265

coptis, 144, 306, 328

corn silk, 286–288, 297,
300, 322

diarrhea, 33, 52, 56, 59, 65, 69–71, 157, 161, 162, 182, 218, 230, 311, 316

digestion, 31, 36, 38, 47, 49–51, 53, 54, 56–61, 63, 64, 66–68, 71, 72, 75, 76, 79, 85, 87, 97, 102, 105, 114, 131, 138, 140, 145, 157, 158, 161, 162, 165, 170, 171, 177, 183–188, 198, 200, 201, 203, 209, 221, 233, 238–240, 245, 256, 259, 262–265, 267, 271, 281, 295, 296, 298, 299, 305, 307, 310, 314, 316, 318, 322

dill, 58, 60, 67, 68, 112, 223, 225, 245, 268, 299, 301, 322

*Dioscorea villosa*
See wild yam

diuretic, 19, 39, 79, 81, 82, 84, 85, 190, 230, 272–274, 283, 285–287, 300

diverticulitis, 52, 65–67, 71

dong quai, 183, 184, 216, 217, 239, 252

dopamine, 124, 125, 128, 135, 260, 261

dry skin, 200–202

dysmenorrhea, 182, 216, 218–220, 230, 317

# E

echinacea, 31, 35, 39, 56, 65, 99, 102, 104, 107, 155, 160, 165, 167, 168, 172, 275, 297, 299, 319, 322, 327

*Echinacea* spp.
See echinacea

Eclectic, 272

eczema, 50, 54, 107, 157, 186–189, 191, 192

elder leaf, 194, 200, 243

elderberry, 107, 108, 112, 116, 167–169, 171, 176, 268, 297, 300, 323

elderflower, 35, 81, 107, 108, 161, 168, 194, 197, 202, 268, 269, 297, 300, 323

elecampane, 105, 111, 113, 114, 116, 157, 298, 323

eleuthero, 131, 133, 134, 136, 175, 176, 180, 214, 255, 262, 263, 266, 275, 276, 278, 296, 320, 321

*Eleutherococcus senticosis*
See eleuthero

embolism, 82, 90, 299

emmenagogue, 83, 215–218, 221, 240, 252, 296, 300

emphysema, 110, 111, 114

endometriosis, 182, 216

Epstein-Barr, 164

erectile dysfunction, 274–276

*Eriodictyon californicum*
See yerba santa

estrogen, 203, 213, 214, 227–229, 232, 239, 250–253, 255

eucalyptus, 107, 114, 157, 159, 163, 166, 180, 297

*Eucalyptus globulus*
See eucalyptus

Euell Gibbons, 17

*Euphrasia* spp.
See eyebright

Eustace Conway, 26

*Eutrochium purpureum*
See Joe Pye weed

evening primrose, 76, 230–232, 242

expectorant, 105, 110, 112–115, 298, 300

exquisite formulary, 26

eyebright, 99, 105, 327

**F**

fatigue, 36, 58, 59, 127, 131, 132, 164, 175, 176, 220, 221, 228, 232, 240, 246, 251, 252, 255, 264, 278

fennel, 20, 58, 60, 62, 67–69, 163, 223, 225, 238, 245, 268, 299, 301, 322

fenugreek, 60, 68, 69, 301

feverfew, 37, 97, 168, 194, 219, 231, 257

fiber, 34, 51–53, 59, 65, 66, 71

fibroids, 182, 183, 213, 216, 225, 231–234

*Filipendula ulmaria*
See meadowsweet

flax, 76, 253, 308

*Foeniculum vulgare*
See fennel

follicle stimulating hormone, 213, 227

foxglove, 78, 309

# G

GABA, 130, 132, 251

galactagogues, 245, 301

Galen, 16, 20, 121

*Gallium aparine*
See cleavers

gallstones, 87

garlic, 29, 31, 39, 53, 68, 76, 82, 86, 88, 89, 91, 92, 102, 104, 106–108, 111, 112, 159, 162, 163, 167, 171, 204, 275–277, 285, 288, 297, 299, 300, 323

gas, 52, 67, 245

gentian, 41, 56, 201, 297–299, 328

*Geranium maculatum*
See cranesbill

giardia, 161–163

Gilgamesh, 15

ginger, 29, 31, 36, 41, 42, 53, 60, 67–69, 71, 72, 81, 86, 92, 97, 101, 107, 140, 170, 176, 179, 183, 184, 191, 201, 202, 216, 218–220, 225, 239, 241, 246, 254, 265, 266, 273, 275, 277–279, 297, 299, 300, 322

ginkgo, 27, 35, 37, 80–82, 89, 92, 97, 104, 136, 139, 140, 144, 145, 147, 176, 198, 202, 219, 231, 257, 267, 279, 302, 314–316, 320, 321, 323

*Ginkgo biloba*
See ginkgo

ginseng, 31, 144, 155, 166, 167, 175, 214, 254, 255, 262, 275, 277, 278, 296, 302, 321, 325, 327

*Glycine max*
See soy

glycoside, 78, 302, 308, 309

*Glycyrrhiza glabra*
See licorice

goddesses, 14, 250

goldenseal, 35, 39, 62, 99, 102, 105–107, 111, 144, 155, 157, 163, 170, 172, 196, 197, 245, 297, 298, 302, 306, 327

gotu kola, 27, 97, 104, 139, 144, 145, 198, 201, 231, 235, 275, 279, 314, 315

Graves' disease, 267, 268

green tea, 41, 77, 111, 233, 268, 274, 283, 318, 321

grief, 80, 92–95, 131, 317

griffonia, 128

*Griffonia simplicifoclia*
See griffonia

# H

*Hammamelis virginiana*
See witch hazel

haritaki, 31

harmaline, 125, 126

*Harpagophytum procumbens*
See devil's claw

hawthorn, 27, 35, 42, 78–83, 88, 91, 92, 94, 95, 141, 144, 147, 201, 257, 266–269, 275, 279, 299, 315, 316, 321

hay fever, 105, 314

headache, 37, 49, 53, 56, 58, 95–98, 100, 112, 130, 145, 173, 179, 194, 218, 219, 221, 228, 229, 231, 232, 257, 263

heart attack, 76, 80, 89–91, 318

heart disease, 74–76, 79, 80, 82, 86, 109, 110, 275

heart palpitations, 38, 39, 53, 80, 252, 257, 267, 269

heartache, 92, 93, 95

*Helicobacter pylori*, 50, 62, 64, 88, 158, 159

helonias, 212, 218, 241, 254, 321, 327

henbane, 304

hepatitis, 54–56, 158, 164, 166, 174

hepatotoxic, 130, 301, 307, 314

herpes, 55, 164, 166, 167, 170

hibiscus, 82, 83

*Hibiscus rosa-sinensis*
   See hibiscus

high blood pressure, 64, 81–84, 87, 113, 201, 253

Hippocrates, 16

Hodgkin's lymphoma, 171

holy basil, 27, 31, 94, 97, 130, 133, 134, 180, 214, 263

homeopathy, 6, 20, 178, 241, 301, 304

honey, 20, 31, 60, 94, 95, 194, 195, 301

hops, 68, 181, 198, 242, 247, 252, 254, 256, 257, 296, 303, 314, 322

horehound, 113, 298

hormone modulators, 214, 232

horseradish, 35, 101, 103, 107, 108, 168

horsetail, 34, 223, 238, 314, 315, 320

*Hydrastis canadensis*
   See goldenseal

hyperactivity, 135, 267

hypercholesterolemia, 86, 88

hypertension, 41, 55, 82, 88, 109, 201, 253, 267, 274, 307, 313, 317

hyperthyroidism, 29, 264–269, 316

hypotension, 84–86, 315, 316

hypothyroidism, 33, 264–266, 316

hyssop, 105, 111, 112, 116

# I

IBD
   See inflammatory Bowel Disease

IBS
   See Irritable Bowel Syndrome

*Impatiens capensis*
   See jewelweed

indigestion, 19, 51, 52, 57, 58, 60, 114, 182, 211, 240, 298, 307 infection, 17, 27, 35, 39, 55, 56, 62–67, 70, 71, 81, 96, 100–111, 115, 139, 154, 157–160, 162, 165, 166, 172–175, 186–192, 195, 234, 243, 244, 246, 272, 282–286, 288, 295

infertility, 214, 227, 234–236

Inflammatory Bowel Disease, 58, 59, 61, 67

influenza, 32, 59, 96, 107, 164, 166, 167, 170, 171

insomnia, 19, 42, 67, 130, 131, 135, 178, 181, 198, 199, 219, 228, 241, 251, 252, 256, 257, 302, 313

iodine deficiency disorder, 33

iron, 27, 33, 34, 190, 221, 223, 233, 239, 301, 314–317

irritability, 36, 49, 57, 58, 67, 147, 218, 230, 241, 267

Irritable Bowel Syndrome, 36, 37, 57

## J

Jamaican dogwood, 41, 42, 97, 178, 181, 219, 220, 232, 234, 275, 276, 296

Japanese knotweed, 174, 175

jaundice, 54, 57, 63

jewelweed, 115, 202

Joe Pye weed, 285, 286, 297

John Gerard, 16

Joseph Lister, 17

*Juglans nigra*
See walnut

Juliette de Bairacli Levy, 196

juniper, 166, 285, 286, 304

*Juniperus communis*
See juniper

## K

kava kava, 126, 303, 328

kelp, 29, 41, 221, 233, 264, 316

khella, 92, 111, 115, 116

kichari, 30

kidney stones, 40, 172, 283–285, 315

# M

magnesium, 27, 63, 223, 231, 314–317

maitake, 170, 268

malaria, 33, 161, 306

malnutrition, 32–34

marshmallow, 61, 189, 192, 193, 195, 274

mastic, 64, 82, 88

mastitis, 245, 246

*Matricaria recutita*
See chamomile

meadowsweet, 42, 97, 106, 179, 181, 194, 219, 232, 234, 296, 297

measles, 33, 164

*Melissa officinalis*
See lemon balm

menarche, 209, 211, 212, 225, 251

menopause, 108, 138, 139, 209, 212, 232, 249–255

menorrhagia, 33, 220, 221, 231

*Mentha* × *piperita*
See peppermint

*Mentha spicata*
See spearmint

metal toxicity, 55, 142

migraine, 49, 95, 97

milk thistle, 55–57, 155, 188, 190, 201, 224, 256, 265, 266, 301, 315, 322

Mithridates, 20

monoamine oxidase inhibitor, 125

mononucleosis, 59, 164

morning sickness, 239–241, 297

motherwort, 19, 37, 39, 41, 42, 56, 61, 79, 82, 83, 86, 91, 92, 94, 95, 129–131, 133, 134, 176, 183, 198, 201, 214, 215, 220, 221, 225, 230–235, 242, 247, 256, 257, 262, 263, 266–269, 275, 296–298, 304, 315–317, 321, 322

*Mucuna pruriens*
See velvet bean

mugwort, 162, 217, 298, 304

mullein, 41, 94, 102, 104, 105, 109, 112, 114, 116, 161, 168, 169, 181, 224, 257, 268, 298, 304, 317, 323

multiple sclerosis, 127

mustard, 36, 107, 179, 181, 221, 233, 265, 296, 297, 303, 309

myelin sheath, 126, 127, 146, 251

myrrh, 20, 297

# N

nausea, 53, 63, 65, 84, 86, 100, 112, 140, 178, 179, 198, 219, 239–241, 297, 298

*Nepeta cataria*
See catnip

nervine, 19, 37, 60, 64, 66, 67, 79, 97, 102, 104, 106, 121, 122, 129–131, 137, 139, 141, 177, 183, 187, 193, 198, 201, 214, 219, 229, 232, 235, 240, 242, 247, 256, 262, 263, 275, 278, 283, 295, 296, 298, 302

nervous system herbs, 121, 262

nettle, 27, 34, 35, 38–42, 55, 58, 71, 72, 91, 134, 160, 168, 192, 201, 202, 215, 217, 221–223, 234, 238, 256, 257, 266, 268, 273, 274, 279, 283, 286, 296, 297, 301, 303, 304, 315– 318, 320, 321, 323

neurotransmitters, 124–126, 129, 130, 132, 146

Nicholas Culpeper, 16

*Nigella*
See black cumin

night-blooming cereus, 92

non-Hodgkin's lymphoma, 171

nootropics, 121

noradrenaline, 124, 129, 130, 261

# O

oak, 70, 196, 243, 298, 304, 311

*oat milky tops*
See oats

oats, 27, 34, 52, 58, 66, 71, 80, 83, 86, 88, 91, 92, 98, 133, 134, 136, 141, 180, 202, 214, 222, 223, 231, 235, 247, 254, 256, 262, 263, 275, 278, 300, 320

oatstraw, 27, 34, 35, 58, 71, 80, 83, 86, 88, 91, 180, 195, 198, 202, 221, 233, 238, 275, 314–317

obesity, 32, 74, 75, 82, 274

oligomenorrhea, 216, 235

omega-3 fatty acids, 76, 87, 242

oregano, 52, 68, 76, 77, 111, 112, 157, 159, 163, 196, 197, 265, 285

Oregon grape, 39, 144, 157, 168, 302, 328

osha, 99, 106, 300, 327

**P**

pain, 25, 41, 42, 55, 57, 59, 63–65, 90, 95, 97, 101, 102, 106, 110, 128, 162, 165, 172, 175, 177–180, 182–184, 193, 196–199, 216, 218–220, 230–234, 246, 262, 283, 284, 288, 303, 306

*palliative*
　　See analgesic

*Panax ginseng*
　　See ginseng

panic, 130, 198, 199, 242, 252, 256

*Papaver somniferum*
　　See poppy

parasites, 53, 106, 153, 161, 163, 201, 297

Parkinson's disease, 128, 129, 142, 183

parsley, 20, 41, 112, 221, 230, 233, 287, 298–301

*Passiflora incarnata*
　　See passionflower

passionflower, 37, 65, 67, 96, 126, 130–133, 199, 201, 202, 219, 220, 232, 235, 236, 242, 256, 257, 262, 275, 296

pau d'arco, 40, 111, 159, 160, 175, 189–191

Paul Stamets, 170

pelvic inflammatory disease, 182

pennyroyal, 68, 296, 300

peppermint, 27, 67, 68, 85, 86, 103, 104, 107, 111, 112, 116, 133, 136, 140, 147, 163, 170, 219, 240, 241, 243, 254, 275, 277, 278, 300

periwinkle, 146, 297

*Piper cubeba*
　See cubeb

pipsissewa, 286, 315, 328

*Pistacia lentiscus*
　See mastic

plague, 20

*Plantago major*
　See plantain

plantain, 61, 62, 66, 69, 72, 105, 109, 180, 192, 193, 195, 197, 242, 243, 246, 275, 286, 302, 304

pleurisy, 111, 114

pleurisy root, 99, 112, 116, 161, 300, 328

Pliny the Elder, 20

PMS
　See pre-menstrual syndrome

pneumonia, 33, 110, 114

*Polygonum cuspidatum*
　See Japanese knotweed

polymenorrhea, 216, 235

polypharmacy, 18–20

poppy, 199, 223, 296

post-partum depression, 131, 133, 134, 247

post-partum tissue care, 243

post-traumatic stress disorder, 131, 133

potassium, 27, 34, 63, 82, 126, 223, 287, 315–317

pre-menstrual syndrome, 76, 227, 228

premenstrual dysphoric disorder, 228

prickly ash, 41, 42, 57, 80–82, 86, 91, 92, 160, 171, 180, 201, 265

Priorities for Care, 3, 4

probiotics, 65, 71, 188

progesterone, 203, 213, 220, 227–229, 232, 239, 250–253, 255

rose hips, 53, 87, 88, 91, 167, 169, 268, 323

rosemary, 77, 112, 139, 145, 147, 157, 159, 163, 166, 196, 201, 265, 279

*Rosmarinus officinalis*
See rosemary

rubefacient, 103, 277, 303

rubella, 33, 164

*Rubus ideaus*
See raspberry

*Rubus villosus*
See blackberry

rue, 56, 83, 126, 162, 298, 304

*Ruscus aculeatus*
See butcher's broom

*Ruta graveolens*
See rue

# S

shamanism, 14, 15

sage, 58, 68, 70, 71, 77, 98, 105, 107, 108, 111, 112, 114, 116, 157, 159, 160, 163, 168, 170, 197, 243, 245, 252, 254, 268, 297, 298, 328

*Salvia* spp.
See sage

*Sambucus nigra*
See elderberry

Samuel Hahnemann, 301

Samuel Thomson, 21

saponin, 253

*Sarothamnus scoparius*
See Scotch broom

saw palmetto, 41, 167, 272–275, 283, 317, 321

schisandra, 55, 140, 214, 263, 266, 278

*Schisandra chinensis*
See schisandra

Scotch broom, 84

Scots pine, 180, 181

sedative, 1, 29, 66, 128, 130–132, 178, 179, 183, 198, 199, 241, 242, 263, 266, 277, 298, 303

seizures, 130, 199

Selective Serotonin Reuptake Inhibitor (SSRI), 126

self-heal, 35, 268

senna, 302, 309

*Serenoa repens*
    See saw palmetto

serotonin, 124–126, 132, 139, 140, 319

shatavari, 31

shea butter, 127

shepherd's purse, 70, 105, 196, 221, 232, 234, 243

shiitake, 170, 268

shingles, 164

*Silybum marianum*
    See milk thistle

Simpler's Method, 19

*Simplocarpus foetidus*
    See skunk cabbage

sinus congestion, 35, 100, 105, 108, 115, 140, 168

skullcap, 65, 67, 95, 97, 130, 166, 181, 195, 198, 201, 214, 219, 230–232, 235, 242, 247, 256, 257, 262, 296–298, 314, 320

skunk cabbage, 115

slippery elm, 35–37, 58, 61, 62, 65, 71, 109, 163, 197, 286, 300, 302, 322, 327

soy, 221, 233, 252, 253, 309

spasmolytic
    See antispasmodic

spearmint, 22, 58, 64, 67–69, 77, 85, 91, 94, 140, 170, 219, 221, 225, 240, 241, 254, 268, 278, 299, 322, 323

spilanthes, 169, 175, 268

St. John's wort, 94, 95, 103, 104, 106, 107, 126, 129, 131–134, 197, 235, 243, 254, 262, 269, 275, 296, 298, 299, 304, 319, 320

stephania, 174

Stephen Buhner, 173

stone root, 283, 285, 286, 328

storax, 127

strep throat, 100

stroke, 74, 75, 82, 86, 89, 90, 110, 138, 142

swollen breasts, 228

*Syzygium aromaticum*
   See clove

# T

*Tabebuia impetiginosa*
   See pau d'arco

*Taraxacum vulgare*
   See dandelion

tea tree, 157–159, 163

teasel, 175

testosterone, 86, 203, 214, 252, 274

*Theobroma cacao*
   See cocoa

Theory of Humors, 16

theriac, 20

thrombosis, 80, 88, 89, 299

*Thuja occidentalis*
   See white cedar

thyme, 20, 29, 68, 77, 106, 111, 112, 157, 196, 197, 221, 233, 285, 297, 300

thyroid, 142, 209, 214, 234, 252, 260, 261, 263, 264, 266, 267

*Tilia europa*
   See linden

Traditional Chinese Medicine, 18, 140, 216, 276

transition, 93, 241, 242, 255

Trotula of Salerno, 16

turmeric, 41, 42, 56, 60, 71, 98, 112, 126–129, 133, 146, 147, 155, 179, 183, 201, 234, 246, 273, 275, 301

# U

ulcers, 50, 62–65, 88, 158, 164, 166, 175, 316

*Ulmus fulva*
   See slippery elm

*Uncaria guianensis*
   See cat's claw

United Nations' World Health Organization, 32

United Plant Savers, 27, 99, 106, 157, 212, 245, 325, 326

urinary tract infection, 39, 81, 283, 285, 288

usnea, 286, 297

UTI
See urinary tract infection

uva ursi, 114

# V

valerian, 66, 68, 179, 181, 184, 198, 242, 246, 256, 263, 297, 303, 314

vasoconstrictor, 84

vasodilator, 37, 81, 82, 129, 140, 144, 183

velvet bean, 128, 129

*Verbascum thapsus*
See mullein

vervain, 27, 42, 79, 136, 180, 219, 232, 246, 247, 254, 255, 257, 262, 263, 296, 298, 314, 316, 320

*Viburnum opulus*
See cramp bark

violet, 27, 35, 94, 111, 116, 180, 197, 239, 246, 254, 317, 318, 322

vitamin A, 33, 34

vitamin C, 33, 79, 87, 221, 222, 233, 314, 317, 318

vitamin D, 33, 86, 222

*Vitex agnus-castus*
See chaste tree berry

vulnerary, 36, 139, 196, 243, 244, 277, 304, 311

# W

walnut, 162, 296, 298, 304, 309

warming herbs, 36, 60, 85, 103, 219, 254, 265

white cedar, 115

white poplar, 41

wild cherry, 114, 116, 170

wild indigo, 99, 298, 328

wild lettuce, 303, 320

wild sarsaparilla, 85, 86, 95, 140, 175, 176, 254, 275–278

wild yam, 41, 60, 62, 66–69, 155, 178, 183, 212, 214, 218–221, 225, 230, 232, 234, 239, 253, 254, 287, 297, 299, 320, 327

willow, 41, 97, 106, 179, 181, 194, 199, 219, 232, 246, 296, 308 wintergreen, 41, 68, 103, 180, 286, 296, 297, 309

witch hazel, 62, 70, 163, 164, 179, 196, 224, 243, 298, 311

wormwood, 162, 298, 304

# Y

yarrow, 19, 35, 36, 39, 40, 67, 70, 81, 85, 92, 105, 107, 108, 112, 160, 161, 171, 180, 194, 196, 197, 200, 215, 217, 219, 221, 232, 243, 245, 246, 254, 256, 273, 274, 277–279, 285, 286, 297, 298, 300, 304, 322

yeast, 53, 159, 160, 186–189, 191

yellow dock, 134, 191, 221, 222, 224, 233, 265, 296, 301, 302, 314, 315, 320

yerba santa, 114

yin-yang philosophy, 276

# Z

*Zanthoxylum americanum*
    See prickly ash

*Zingiber officinale*
    See ginger